AIDS

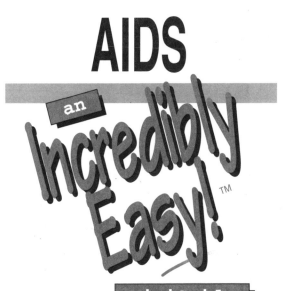

an Incredibly Easy!™

MiniGuide

AIDS

an

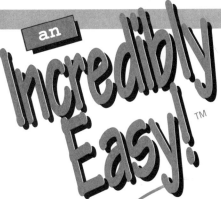

Incredibly Easy!™

MiniGuide

Staff

Vice President
Matthew Cahill

Clinical Director
Judith A. Schilling McCann,
RN, MSN

Art Director
John Hubbard

Executive Editor
Michael Shaw

Managing Editor
Andrew T. McPhee, RN,
BSN

Clinical Editors
Jill M. Curry, RN, BSN,
CCRN; Collette Bishop
Hendler, RN, CCRN; Joan M.
Robinson, RN, MSN, CCRN;
Carla M. Roy, RN, BSN,
CCRN; Gwynn Sinkinson,
RNC, NP

Editor
Kevin Haworth, Edward R.
Pratowski

Copy Editors
Brenna H. Mayer (manager),
Gretchen Fee, Stacey A.
Follin, Pamela Wingrod

Designers
Arlene Putterman (associate art director), Mary
Ludwicki (book designer),
Joseph John Clark, Susan
Sheridan

Illustrators
Bot Roda, Betty Winnberg

Typography
Diane Paluba (manager),
Joyce Rossi Biletz, Valerie
Molettiere

Manufacturing
Deborah Meiris (director),
Patricia K. Dorshaw (manager), Otto Mezei (book production manager)

Editorial Assistants
Beverly Lane, Marcia Mills,
Liz Schaeffer

Indexer
Ellen Murray

The clinical treatments described
and recommended in this publication are based on research and
consultation with nursing, medical,
and legal authorities. To the best of
our knowledge, these procedures
reflect currently accepted practice.
Nevertheless, they can't be considered absolute and universal recommendations. For individual applications, all recommendations must be
considered in light of the patient's
clinical condition and, before
administration of new or infrequently used drugs, in light of the
latest package-insert information.
The authors and the publisher disclaim any responsibility for any
adverse effects resulting from the
suggested procedures, from any
undetected errors, or from the
reader's misunderstanding of the
text.

Printed in the United States of
America.

IEMAIDS-010899

Ⓡ A member of the Reed Elsevier plc group

**Library of Congress Cataloging-in-
Publication Data**

AIDS: an incredibly easy miniguide
     p. cm.
     Includes index.
     1. AIDS (disease) handbooks,
     manuals, etc. 2. AIDS (disease)—
     Nursing handbooks, manuals, etc.
     I. Springhouse Corporation.
RC607.A26A3455514 1999
616.97'92—dc21   99-23043
ISBN 1-58255-014-X (alk. paper) CIP

Contents

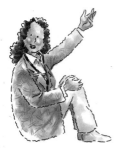

Contributors and consultants

Joanne M. Bartelmo, RN, MSN, CCRN
Clinical Educator
Pottstown (Pa.) Memorial
Medical Center

Michael Carter, RN, DNSc, FAAN
Dean and Professor
College of Nursing
University of Tennessee
Memphis

Nancy Cirone, RN,C, MSN, CDE
Director of Education
Warminster (Pa.) Hospital

Margaret Friant Cramer, RN, MSN
Clinical Supervisor
Cardiac Solutions, Inc.
Fort Washington, Pa.

Pamela Mullen Kovach, RN, BSN
Independent Clinical
Consultant
Perkiomenville, Pa.

Patricia A. Lange, RN, MSN, EdD (candidate), **CS, CCRN**
Graduate Nursing Program
Coordinator and Assistant
Professor of Nursing
Hawaii Pacific University
Kaneohe

Mary Ann Siciliano McLaughlin, RN, MSN
Clinical Supervisor
Cardiac Solutions, Inc.
Fort Washington, Pa.

Lori Musolf Neri, RN, MSN, CCRN
Clinical Instructor
Villanova (Pa.) University
ICU Staff Nurse
North Penn Hospital
Lansdale, Pa.

Joseph L. Neri, DO, FACC
Cardiologist
The Heart Care Group
Allentown, Pa.

Robert Rauch
Manager of Government
Economics
Amgen, Inc.
Thousand Oaks, Calif.

Larry E. Simmons, RN, PhD
(candidate)
Clinical Instructor
University of Missouri-
Kansas City

Foreword

With the help of new treatments and preventive therapies, people with HIV infection and AIDS remain well longer than ever before. The outlook is much more hopeful. However, because of the ability of HIV to mutate readily, hope must be tempered with caution. Health care providers must be as vigilant as ever in fulfilling their role as patient advocates, providing health education for their patients and keeping up-to-date on the latest information about treatments.

No one should underestimate the challenge of providing care for patients with HIV infection and AIDS. That's why the clinical experts at Springhouse decided to create *AIDS: An Incredibly Easy MiniGuide,* a revolutionary new AIDS patient–care reference. Accurate, authoritative, and completely up-to-date, this handy book will help you gain an in-depth understanding of HIV infection and AIDS in an unusually offbeat, uplifting, and easygoing way.

The first chapter, *Understanding AIDS,* lays the foundation for excellent patient care by providing basic facts about the pathophysiology of HIV infection and its effects on the body. The next three chapters cover prevention, assessment, and treatment of HIV infection and AIDS. The fifth chapter covers complications, including opportunistic infections and malignancies such as Kaposi's sarcoma. The final chapter covers patient teaching.

Throughout the book, you'll find special features designed to strengthen your understanding of HIV infection and AIDS. For instance, *Memory joggers* provide clever tricks for remembering key points. *Checklists,* rendered in the style of a classroom chalkboard, provide at-a-glance summaries of important facts.

Cartoon characters appear throughout to provide lighthearted chuckles as well as reinforcement of essential material. And a *Quick quiz* at the end of every chapter gives you a chance to assess your learning and refresh your memory at the same time.

The depth of information contained in this truly pocket-size guide will impress even the most experienced health care professional. If you want an easy-to-read, comprehensive reference about one of today's most important health care challenges, I can't think of a better resource than *AIDS: An Incredibly Easy MiniGuide*. It packs a wallop.

Michael Carter, RN, DNSc, FAAN
Dean and Professor
College of Nursing
University of Tennessee
Memphis

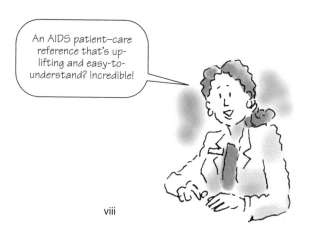

An AIDS patient–care reference that's up-lifting and easy-to-understand? Incredible!

Understanding AIDS

Key facts
◆ AIDS results from infection with human immunodeficiency virus, a retrovirus.

◆ To date, five types of retrovirus have been identified.

◆ In AIDS, a patient is more susceptible to certain opportunistic infections and diseases.

About AIDS

AIDS, which stands for acquired immunodeficiency syndrome, is now the 17th leading cause of mortality in the United States. AIDS is actually a collection of conditions in which a markedly weakened immune system plays a key role. Severe immunodeficiency results in susceptibility to numerous opportunistic infections and diseases. The appearance of these opportunistic infections and diseases signals AIDS.

I attack cells in the immune system, leaving patients susceptible to infection and disease.

HIV vs. the immune system

This condition is caused by human immuno-deficiency virus (HIV), a retrovirus that attacks certain cells in the immune system and ultimately destroys them.

Nothing definitive

There is no definitive list of symptoms for AIDS. However, AIDS is usually signaled by suppressed immune status and the onset of opportunistic infections.

History of AIDS

The Centers for Disease Control and Prevention first described the syndrome that came to be known as AIDS in 1981. This syndrome initially appeared among a group of young men suffering from unusual cancers and rare opportunistic diseases. Researchers at the National Institutes of Health and other infectious disease centers began searching for the cause of this "new" disease.

Searching for answers

At first, researchers labeled AIDS a vene-real disease because the majority of cases occurred among homosexual men. In the early and mid-1980s, substantial epidemiological research focused on a homosexual man from Canada thought to have brought HIV to the United States from abroad.

Although this one man may have introduced HIV to several communities, scientists now know that the virus has existed in humans since 1959 and possibly before.

Eureka!

Eureka!

In 1983, scientists isolated a retrovirus and named it human immunodeficiency virus (HIV). One of the deadliest retroviruses found in humans, HIV is transmitted by blood and body secretions. The virus also causes disease in such animals as sheep, monkeys, goats, and cattle.

A proven relationship

HIV ultimately leads to AIDS, the final stage in HIV infection. (See *Understanding an AIDS diagnosis,* page 5.) Scientists proved the relationship between HIV and AIDS in 1984. The most common form of HIV, a virus now known as HIV-1, was identified in 1984. Another form, HIV-2, was discovered in West Africa in 1986. Soon after, testing methods were developed.

Pan troglodytes and sooty mangabeys

Current evidence suggests that HIV-1 first appeared in chimpanzees called *pan troglodytes* and that HIV-2 first appeared in monkeys called *sooty mangabeys.* Research into the structure of early forms of HIV may help scientists to understand how the virus mutated into the forms seen today. Understanding those mutations may, in turn, lead to better testing and treatment methods.

Pathophysiology of AIDS

To understand what happens in AIDS, consider the pathophysiology of viruses and retroviruses.

Viruses

Viruses come in a number of shapes but all are constructed from arrays of protein pieces. Inside a virus's outer protein layer is little more than the deoxyribonucleic acid (DNA) or ribonucleic acid (RNA) the virus needs to copy itself.

Now I get it!

Understanding an AIDS diagnosis

According to the Centers for Disease Control and Prevention (CDC), the following three conditions must be met to establish a diagnosis of AIDS:

🖐 presence of HIV infection

✌ CD4+ cell (T-cell) count of fewer than 200/μl

🖐 presence of one or more conditions specified by the CDC. (These conditions are divided into categories A, B, and C. For a list of these conditions, see the appendix, Conditions that define AIDS.)

Retroviruses

HIV is a type of virus known as a retrovirus. Retroviruses infect a cell and then integrate their own genetic material into the cell's DNA, forever changing the DNA of the host cell. As soon as retroviruses change the DNA of a host cell, they use the cell's RNA to build a sort of virus factory within the cell.

HIV mainly targets two types of white blood cell: macrophages and T cells. Of the T cells, a type of T cell called a helper

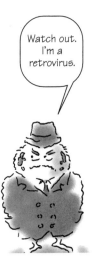

Watch out. I'm a retrovirus.

T cell, or CD4$^+$ cell, is particularly vulnerable to HIV. (See *Immune system cells*.)

1 into 250

A single HIV particle in a macrophage or T cell can prompt its host to make as many as 250 new virus particles before destroying the cell.

Effects of HIV

After HIV has invaded a host cell, the host cell produces more virus particles every

(Text continues on page 17.)

One of me can multiply into as many as 250 virus particles.

Now I get it!

Immune system cells

The immune system has two primary types of cells: lymphocytes (or lymphoid cells) and nonlymphoid cells.

Lymphocytes

Lymphocytes help defend the body against fungi, viruses, protozoa, and certain intracellular bacteria. They're divided into two types: B cells and T cells.

- B cells change into plasma cells and secrete antibodies. B-cell immune responses are called humoral immunity.
- T cells are responsible for the immune responses known as cell-mediated immunity. Two T-cell groups come into play in HIV infection: T4 cells and T8 cells. T4 cells (also known as CD4+ cells or helper T cells) enhance the immune response. These cells are especially vulnerable to HIV. T8 cells (CD8+ cells, or suppressor T cells) inhibit the immune response.

(continued)

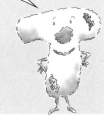

My job is to produce antibodies that will attack an antigen.

In cell-mediated immunity, I attack the antigen directly.

Immune system cells (continued)

Nonlymphoid cells

Nonlymphoid cells are phagocytic cells (capable of ingesting particulate matter). They include neutrophils (granulocytes) and macrophages.

• Neutrophils, the most common type of granulocyte, provide the body's main defense against bacteria and other extracellular pathogens. HIV doesn't seem to infect these cells.

• Macrophages are derived from monocytes, a type of leukocyte (white blood cell). Macrophages change into active, aggressive cells within host tissues. Then they phagocytose foreign substances and kill them. Recent studies indicate that HIV infects macrophages.

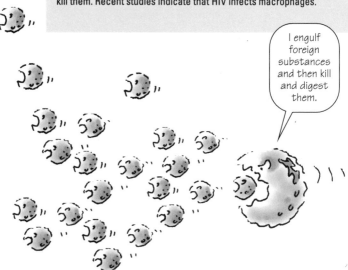

How a virus infects a cell

In many ways, HIV infects cells the way other viruses do. The next four illustrations show how a typical virus infects a cell.

Attaching to the host cell

The virus attaches to a host cell, opens, and injects its genetic material (deoxyribonucleic acid [DNA] or ribonucleic acid [RNA]) into the host cell.

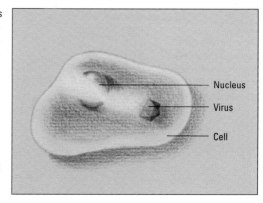

Nucleus

Virus

Cell

Copying the viral genome

The virus uses the host cell's metabolic and reproductive capacity to make copies of the viral genome, the virus's complete DNA or RNA strand. All of the genetic material needed to replicate the virus is contained in the host cell.

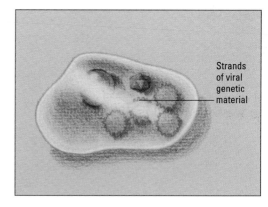

Strands of viral genetic material

How a virus infects a cell *(continued)*

Making the protein shell

The virus then directs the host cell to make a protein shell for each viral genome, thereby creating a new virus.

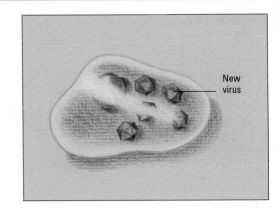

New virus

Releasing new viruses

The cell releases new viruses. New viruses go on to infect other cells. Release of the new viruses generally causes destruction of the host cell.

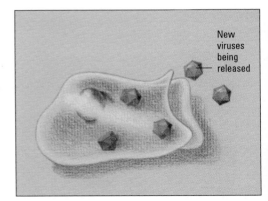

New viruses being released

Structure of HIV

The ability of HIV to infect a wide variety of cells — from T cells to B cells to endothelial and epithelial cells — stems in part from its structure as well as its ability to mutate. This illustration shows the key components of an HIV particle.

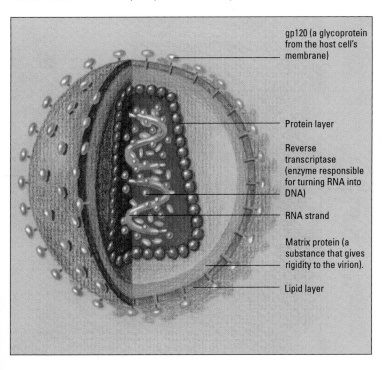

gp120 (a glycoprotein from the host cell's membrane)

Protein layer

Reverse transcriptase (enzyme responsible for turning RNA into DNA)

RNA strand

Matrix protein (a substance that gives rigidity to the virion).

Lipid layer

How HIV attaches to a cell

HIV primarily infects T-cell lymphocytes and macrophages, key components of the immune system. To infect a cell, the virus must first attach itself to the host cell's outer membrane. The attachment of gp120 (a glycoprotein) to the T cell's CD4+ receptor site allows gp41 (another glycoprotein) to start virus-to-cell membrane fusion. This illustration shows how that attachment occurs.

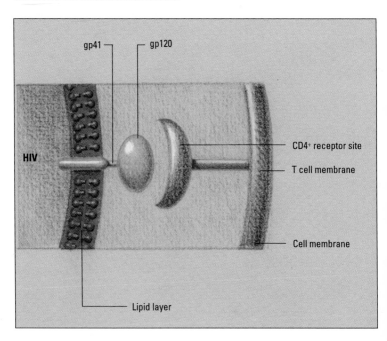

How HIV takes over a cell

HIV takes over each cell it invades and uses the cell's own components to do it — the hallmark characteristic of a retrovirus. These illustrations show how HIV enters and takes over a cell.

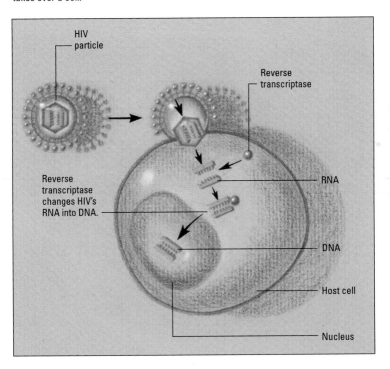

How HIV takes over a cell *(continued)*

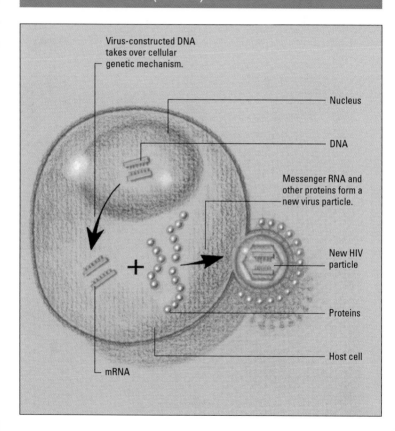

Diseases caused by HIV infection

A wide variety of opportunistic diseases occur among patients with AIDS or HIV infection. These photos show a few of the more common of those diseases.

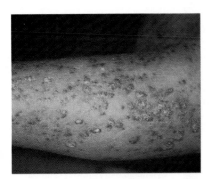

Kaposi's sarcoma lesions
The most common AIDS-related cancer, Kaposi's sarcoma is characterized by obvious, colorful lesions, shown at left. The disease causes structural and functional damage. When associated with AIDS, it progresses aggressively, involving the lymph nodes, viscera and, possibly, GI structures.

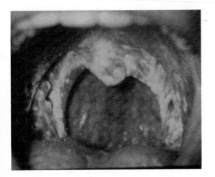

Candidiasis (thrush)
Candidiasis of the oropharyngeal mucosa (thrush) causes cream-colored or bluish white pseudomembranous patches on the tongue, oral mucosa, or pharynx, shown at left. Fungal invasion may extend to circumoral tissues.

Diseases caused by HIV infection *(continued)*

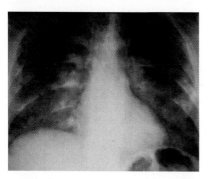

Pneumocystis carinii pneumonia (PCP)

This color-enhanced X-ray (left) shows signs of pneumonia caused by *Pneumocystis carinii*. The diagnosis of PCP can also be made by examination of a first-morning sputum specimen.

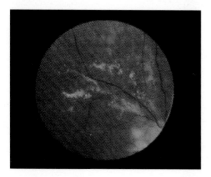

Cytomegalovirus (CMV) retinitis

CMV retinitis is the most common eye disorder in patients with AIDS and may progress rapidly to blindness. Damage caused by the virus results in impaired blood supply. The white cotton-woollike areas in this photo (left) of the eye ground are patches of fatty exudates due to low blood flow to the area.

time it tries to replicate. As T cells decrease in number, the body loses its ability to fight infection, allowing opportunistic infection and disease to occur.

Fungal, viral, protozoal, or bacterial

Opportunistic infections may be fungal in origin (histoplasmosis, candidiasis), viral (cytomegalovirus, herpes), protozoal (*Pneumocystis carinii* pneumonia, toxoplasmosis), or bacterial (tuberculosis, salmonellosis).

Five partners in crime

HIV isn't the only retrovirus of its kind in existence. It's actually one of several retroviruses classified as human T-cell leukemia-lymphoma viruses (HTLV). Each type of HTLV attaches to specialized T cells.

Currently, five types of HTLV have been identified:

• HTLV-I causes adult T-cell leukemia-lymphoma, a cancer of the blood and bone marrow

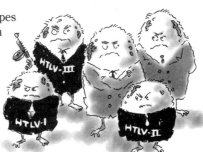

cells. Experts believe HTLV-I, which is transmitted sexually and through sharing infected needles, is related to HIV.

• HTLV-II is associated with hairy cell leukemia.

• HTLV-III, also known as HIV or HIV-1, was the first member of the HTLV family to be linked to AIDS. It was formerly known as lymphadenopathy-associated virus (LAV).

• HTLV-IV, also known as HIV-2 and formerly as LAV-2, also causes AIDS. Although HTLV-IV differs genetically from HTLV-III (HIV-1), it attacks the body in similar ways and causes similar reactions. This virus is most prevalent in Africa.

• HTLV-V, recently discovered in a patient with cutaneous T-cell lymphoma, is a human retrovirus with greater immunosuppression activity than HTLV-I but less than HTLV-III (HIV-1).

An indirect killer

HIV itself doesn't kill its host but instead disables and ultimately destroys the immune system. When that happens, opportunistic infections and other diseases can overrun the body's defenses.

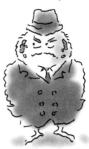

I work slowly, but I wreak havoc on the immune system.

Quick quiz

1. The two HTL viruses known to cause AIDS are:
- A. HTLV-I and HTLV-II.
- B. HTLV-II and HTLV-III.
- C. HTLV-III and HTLV-IV.

Answer: C. HTLV-III and its relative HTLV-IV are now commonly known as HIV-1 and HIV-2. Although these viruses differ genetically, both attack the body in similar ways and both are associated with AIDS.

2. HIV possesses numerous characteristics, including:
- A. long incubation period.
- B. ability to directly cause neoplasm.
- C. transmission through respiratory particles.

Answer: A. HIV can have an extremely long incubation period.

3. The CDC definition of AIDS requires the presence of a CD4+ cell count of:
- A. under 200/μl.
- B. under 500/μl.
- C. above 500/μl.

Answer: A. According to the CDC, a CD4+ cell count under 200/μl is required for a diagnosis of AIDS.

Scoring

☆☆☆ If you answered all three questions correctly, congratulations! Just as a healthy T-cell attacks an antigen, so you have attacked this chapter.

☆☆ If you answered two questions correctly, excellent! You have digested the material in this chapter the way a macrophage digests a foreign substance.

☆ If you answered fewer than two questions correctly, don't fret. Be opportunistic; become reacquainted with this chapter.

2

Preventing AIDS

Key facts
- New cases of HIV infection in the United States increasingly occur among minorities and poor people.
- The primary methods of HIV transmission are sex with an infected partner, contact with infected blood or blood products, and contact between a mother and her infant during the perinatal period.
- Heterosexual sex is the most prevalent method of HIV transmission worldwide.
- Health education and precautions are the only methods currently available to stop HIV transmission.
- Development of a vaccine against HIV may be possible, but scientists must first overcome the mutation and resistance factors of HIV.

AIDS in the United States

In the United States, HIV infection must be reported to the Centers for Disease Control and Prevention (CDC) only when

Ethnic distribution

The chart below shows the ethnic distribution of AIDS cases in the United States.

Population	Percentage of AIDS cases
White	45%
Black, not Hispanic	36%
Hispanic	18%
Asian or Pacific Islander	less than 1%
Native American or Alaskan Native	less than 1%

Source: *Scientific American,* July 1998

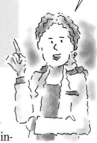

The number of reported AIDS cases reflects only a small percentage of the people infected with HIV.

a diagnosis of AIDS is made. Thus, the number of reported AIDS cases reflects only a small percentage of the people infected with HIV and doesn't account for individuals who might otherwise be diagnosed with AIDS but who haven't been tested for HIV antibodies. Some researchers estimate that for every reported case of AIDS, 50 to 75 people are infected with HIV.

A chronic condition

With the advent of more successful treatment strategies, AIDS is becoming a chronic illness. People are living longer with HIV and AIDS, but HIV infection remains a lifelong condition.

Poor patients, expensive treatments

Unfortunately, AIDS is becoming increasingly prevalent among poor people. Lack of access to health care, social services, and information on preventive guidelines as well as other factors make poor people vulnerable to infection. Many patients lack the skills and resources to demand proper care and can't afford to spend an estimated $10,000 to $20,000 per year on medications and treatments.

Populations at risk

Recent reports from the CDC indicate that nearly 50% of newly diagnosed cases of HIV infection are found among blacks, a population that makes up only 13% of the total U.S. population. The fastest rate of growth is among black women, most of whom acquire the virus through heterosexual contact. Many are impoverished mothers.

Hispanics make up 10% of the U.S. population but 20% of the new AIDS cases. (See *Ethnic distribution*.)

AIDS around the world

HIV infection constitutes a global epidemic. The World Health Organization (WHO) estimates that 40 to 100 million people worldwide may be HIV-infected.

However, no set of numbers for this infection can be considered fully reliable because of:
• lack of testing mechanisms in developing countries
• inability to detect those with early infection (window period)
• cost of testing
• fear of test results
• incomplete statistical reporting, especially in developing countries.

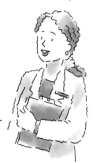

The lack of effective testing makes global HIV estimates unreliable.

European cases expected to decline....

The spread of HIV and the number of AIDS cases in Europe have followed patterns similar to those of the United States. A decline is expected in both areas.

...but cases in Africa are exploding

AIDS most likely originated in Africa, and that continent has been hardest hit by the

HIV-infection and AIDS worldwide

The chart below shows estimates for adult infection with HIV and AIDS worldwide.

Region	AIDS-HIV infection estimate
Australia and New Zealand	12,000
Eastern Europe and Central Asia	150,000
North Africa and Middle East	210,000
Caribbean	310,000
East Asia and Pacific Islands	440,000
Western Europe	530,000
United States	750,000
South America	1.3 million
South and Southeast Asia	6 million
Sub-Saharan Africa	20.8 million
GLOBAL TOTAL	30.5 MILLION

Source: *Scientific American,* July 1998

epidemic. Some regions have reported infection rates estimated at greater than half the population. Like Africa, Asia and South America are now experiencing steady increases in HIV infection. (See *HIV-infection and AIDS worldwide.*)

Transmission

Researchers have isolated HIV in blood, semen, vaginal secretions, breast milk, tears, urine, cerebrospinal fluid, alveolar fluid, and brain tissue. All of these fluids and tissue can contain the virus, but there is no evidence that they all can transmit the virus.

Currently, scientists believe that HIV is transmitted in three ways, through:

 contact with infected blood

sex with an infected partner

contact between a mother and her infant during the perinatal period.

Blood-borne

Blood-borne transmission occurs through:
• accidental needle sticks or sharing of contaminated needles (I.V. drug use is a common source of HIV transmission.)
• transfusion of contaminated blood or blood products
• exposure through an open wound or mucous membrane.

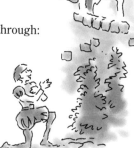

Wait a minute... sexual contact is the most common method of HIV transmission.

Sexual

Sexual contact is the most common method of HIV transmission. Transmission may occur during:

• homosexual sex. About half of the newly diagnosed cases in the United States involve homosexual or bisexual men.

• heterosexual sex. In most cases, transmission occurs from an infected male to an uninfected female, although the opposite may occur.

Mother-to-child

An infected mother can pass HIV to her fetus during pregnancy or to her baby through blood contact during delivery. Postnatally, she may also transmit HIV to her baby through infected breast milk.

> If found, a vaccine would be more cost-effective than current treatments. However, new problems would arise.

Prevention

Developing a vaccine to prevent HIV infection is a major goal in the fight against AIDS. If found, a vaccine would be more cost effective than currently available treatments. Vaccine development, however, poses its own set of problems:

• HIV quickly and readily mutates. As a result, one vaccine may prevent only some subtypes of the infection, much like the current influenza vaccine. Other subtypes would continue to cause infection.

• A vaccine might result in the development of new HIV subtypes or subtypes highly resistant to current therapy.

• A vaccine may provide false assurances of protection. As a result, people may become less diligent about avoiding high risk behaviors.

• Conducting clinical trials for a vaccine may create ethical conflicts.

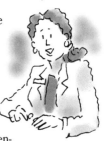

Health education, health promotion activities, and information are the best ways to fight against AIDS.

Primary prevention

Because no vaccine exists to prevent HIV infection and no cure for AIDS exists, primary prevention is the most reliable method for stopping transmission of the virus. Primary prevention includes all interventions that promote health and prevent HIV infection.

Common methods of primary prevention include:

• general health education
• health promotion activities
• information on contraception

• ready availability of protective devices such as condoms.

What to do, exactly

Specific activities to prevent HIV infection include:

• practicing sexual abstinence
• having a mutually monogamous sexual relationship with a person known to be HIV-negative
• practicing safer, protected sex
• refraining from sex with HIV-infected individuals or those at high risk for contracting the virus
• avoiding sexual practices, such as anal sex, that may damage body tissue
• avoiding I.V. drug use
• in artificial insemination, requiring the donor to test HIV-negative twice with 6-month intervals
• donating your own blood for surgery whenever possible
• refraining from sharing toothbrushes, razors, or other personal items that may contain blood or body secretions
• refraining from donating blood if engaged in any high risk behaviors
• undergoing an HIV antibody test if considering pregnancy

Advice from the experts

Advocating safer sex

One way to advocate safer sex is to recommend patients practice sexual behaviors in which they avoid sharing body secretions. Such behaviors include:

- body massage
- closed-mouth kissing
- hugging
- mutual masturbation.

Create a barrier

Patients can lessen the risk of other sexual activities with consistent use of a barrier, such as latex condoms and a spermicide containing nonoxynol-9. In recent studies, nonoxynol-9 has been shown to either inactivate or destroy HIV.

Teach the patient that, because condoms can break, using nonoxynol-9 is important for enhancing protection.

Be leery of lubricants

The patient should never combine oil-based lubricants with latex condoms. Oil-based lubricants increase the risk of condom breakage.

Know the risks

Make sure the patient is aware that all risks can't be eliminated by safer sex precautions.

> Never combine oil-based lubricants with latex condoms.

• providing age-appropriate information to others about safer sex. (See *Advocating safer sex*.)

Especially for health care professionals

Most cases of occupational HIV transmission involving health care professionals have occurred among nurses (55), followed by clinical laboratory technicians (32), nonsurgical physicians (17), health aides (15), and housekeepers and maintenance workers (13).

Here are some primary prevention methods specifically for nurses and other health care personnel:

• Use standard precautions at all times.
• Wash hands regularly.
• Handle all sharps with extreme care.
• Use puncture-resistant containers for sharps disposal.
• Don't re-cap needles.
• Keep emergency ventilatory equipment ready for unexpected circumstances such as cardiopulmonary resuscitation, to avoid the need for mouth-to-mouth resuscitation.

A one-time exposure to HIV-infected blood has an estimated 1-in-300 chance of leading to HIV infection. Comparatively, a

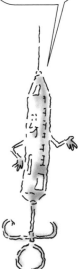

If you think you've been exposed...

If you've been exposed to fluids potentially contaminated with HIV, you should take these steps.

Remove, protect, notify, and reduce

• Attempt to remove as much of the fluid as possible by flushing with water or washing with soap and water. Don't squeeze a puncture site or wound; this may force a virus particle directly into the bloodstream.

• Make sure the patient and others are protected against exposure.

• Notify your immediate supervisor, and follow your facility's policies and procedures. Depending on the size of your facility, you may need to go to the occupational health office or the emergency department.

• Reduce your risk of HIV infection by taking prophylactic antiviral drugs within 2 hours of the incident.

Request, consider, follow, and be proactive

• Request consent for HIV and hepatitis testing from the patient whose body fluids you were exposed to. You should also establish your own HIV and hepatitis status.

• Consider undergoing counseling while waiting for the outcome of your 3-month follow-up testing. Follow-up is essential for your health and well-being.

• Always follow guidelines for safer sex.

• Don't be embarrassed about the incident. Be proactive to protect your own health and safety.

single exposure to hepatitis B has about a 1-in-3 chance of transmission. (See *If you think you've been exposed....*)

Secondary prevention

Secondary prevention of AIDS focuses on early detection of HIV infection and early treatment. Identifying patients at an early stage of infection may help to decrease the severity of illness.

Common interventions at the secondary prevention level include screening activities and education about how to recognize symptoms and reduce the risk of pathologic changes.

Secondary prevention focuses on early detection of HIV infection.

Your patient tests positive. Now what?

If an individual tests positive for HIV, secondary prevention measures include:

• following primary prevention measures
• protecting partners from body secretions during sexual activity
• refraining from donating tissue or blood
• seeking professional help to terminate drug abuse, if applicable
• refraining from sharing drug equipment if unwilling to stop drug abuse
• seeking early treatment of HIV
• informing primary medical provider of HIV status
• notifying former and current sexual

partners so they can be tested for HIV
• cleaning spilled blood or body secretions with 1:10 diluted bleach in water
• avoiding pregnancy
• informing health care workers on a need-to-know basis only, to maintain confidentiality about this highly sensitive issue.

Quick quiz

1. Body secretions not considered a high risk for transmitting HIV include:
  A. blood.
  B. saliva.
  C. semen.
Answer: B. Saliva contains low numbers of virus particles. No evidence to date suggests that saliva can transmit HIV in the absence of bleeding.

2. Primary prevention measures for HIV infection don't include:
  A. having a vasectomy or tubal ligation.
  B. donating your own blood for surgery.
  C. sharing I.V. drug needles only with individuals who test negative for HIV antibodies.

Answer: A. Vasectomies and tubal ligations may prevent pregnancy, but they won't stop HIV transmission.

3. In the United States, the population with the fastest rate of growth for newly diagnosed cases of HIV infection is:
   A.   homosexual or bisexual men.
   B.   black women.
   C.   Hispanic women.

Answer: B. Black women currently have the fastest rate of growth for new cases of HIV infection.

4. If a patient tests positive for HIV, he should do all of the following except:
   A.   notify current and former sexual partners so they can be tested for HIV.
   B.   protect partners from body secretions during sexual activity, especially by using oil-based lubricants with latex condoms.
   C.   seek professional help to terminate drug abuse or refrain from sharing drug equipment if unwilling to stop abuse.

Answer: B. The patient should never combine oil-based lubricants with latex condoms. Oil-based lubricants increase the risk of condom leakage.

Scoring

☆☆ If you answered three or more questions correctly, excellent! You've exposed yourself to solid learning.

☆ If you answered fewer than three questions correctly, take heart. Consider this quiz a preventive measure.

3

Assessing patients with AIDS

Key facts
- An HIV antibody test reveals HIV status 3 months prior to the test, *not* current HIV status.
- HIV testing requires a signed consent form and pretest counseling.
- HIV has a long incubation period — an average of 10 years for an adult, 17 months for children — before it progresses to AIDS.
- Evaluating patients with HIV infection involves assessing opportunistic infections and malignancies.
- HIV infection can affect almost every body system.

AIDS assessment challenge

AIDS offers many assessment challenges. Initially, it may be difficult to diagnose HIV infection because the virus has a long incubation period. Tests may not detect its presence for several months. In addition, signs and symptoms of early HIV infection are often mistaken for the flu.

A 3- to 6-month window

Testing for HIV is inconclusive if antibody formation has yet to occur. The period of infection without antibodies is often described as the "window period" and may last days to months. For the majority of infected people, the window period lasts less than 3 months. For some, it can last longer but usually not more than 6 months. (See *Through the window.*)

From infection to chronic illness

The average time interval between infection and the first signs of AIDS is about 10 years. This figure is based on people who acquired the disease before aggressive multidrug therapy became available and is expected to increase as more HIV-positive individuals receive multidrug therapy.

This 10-year period applies only to adults. For children, the latent period averages about 17 months.

The average time interval before a patient shows signs of AIDS is about 10 years.

Diagnostic tests

Through the window

The window period is the time between the transmission of HIV and the detection of HIV antibodies through testing. If a person is tested for HIV antibodies during this window, the test will come back negative. Most often, the window period lasts 3 months. Cases of conversion after 35 months are rare but have been documented.

Why the window is risky

The window period creates the following health risks:

• Test results may be misleading if a patient exposed to HIV doesn't have a detectable response when the test is administered.
• The patient may develop a false belief that he is uninfected.
• The patient, believing himself free from the virus, may infect others during the window period.

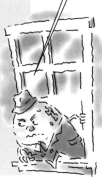

It's difficult to catch me sneaking through the window.

Check everywhere

When assessing a patient with possible HIV infection, you need to thoroughly evaluate his history, physical examination, and diagnostic tests. HIV can indirectly affect almost every body system.

First subtle, then complex

In its early stages, HIV infection tends to produce subtle and nonspecific changes in the body. In later stages, it produces increasingly complex and wide-ranging infections and diseases.

Recognizing acute infection

As the patient develops AIDS, he may display such signs and symptoms as:
- aches and pains in bones and muscles
- anorexia and weight loss
- fever
- headache
- herpetic outbreak
- lymph node enlargement

Memory jogger

To help you remember the general pattern of HIV disease progression, learn the following rhyme:

As HIV progresses

Signs are ever-changing

First they're vague and subtle

Then complex and wide-ranging

- malaise
- nausea, vomiting, and diarrhea
- sore throat.

Marking the progress of HIV infection

You can mark the progress of HIV infection and its progression to AIDS using different systems, including:

- Walter Reed system
- Centers for Disease Control and Prevention system. (See *Classifying HIV disease*, pages 43 to 45.)

Taking the patient's history

Describing HIV-related complaints may be difficult for some patients, especially if they haven't yet been diagnosed. When taking a history, provide emotional support and encourage the patient to openly discuss his condition.

Chief complaint

In its early stages, HIV infection may produce a variety of nonspecific complaints. A patient may complain of any of the following symptoms:

- anorexia
- depression

- diarrhea
- dyspnea on exertion
- fatigue
- fever
- lethargy
- night sweats
- weight loss.

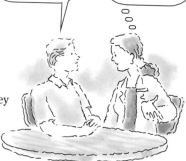

Keep in mind that some patients remain asymptomatic until they abruptly develop *Pneumocystis carinii* pneumonia, a Kaposi's sarcoma lesion, or symptoms of another opportunistic disease.

History of present illness

Explore the patient's chief complaint and other associated complaints. Find out specifics about his symptoms, including:

- when they began
- how long they've lasted
- how severe they seem
- where they're located
- what factors alleviate or precipitate them.

(Text continues on page 45.)

Classifying HIV disease

The two major classification systems for staging HIV disease are the Walter Reed Staging and Classification System and the Centers for Disease Control and Prevention (CDC) system. Each system stages the progress of HIV disease according to a different set of criteria.

Walter Reed Staging and Classification System

Walter Reed Staging and Classification System is a seven-stage system for classifying stages of HIV disease. Stages of illness are based on the presence of HIV antibodies, chronic lymphadenopathy, $CD4^+$ cell counts, skin testing, and the presence of thrush or other opportunistic infections.

Stage	Description
WR0	Negative for HIV antibodies, absence of chronic lymphadenopathy, $CD4^+$ cell count over 400, a normal reaction to skin testing, and the absence of thrush or other opportunistic infections
WR1	The same as WR0 except positive for HIV antibodies
WR2	The same as WR0 except positive for HIV antibodies and presence of chronic lymphadenopathy
WR3	The same as WR0 except positive for HIV antibodies and a $CD4^+$ cell count under 400. (Chronic lymphadenopathy may not exist at this stage.)
WR4	The same as WR3 with a partial defect in skin testing
WR5	The same as WR3 with anergy on skin testing or thrush present
WR6	The same as WR3 with the presence of thrush and one or more opportunistic infections. (Skin testing may produce normal anergy results at this stage.)

Classifying HIV disease *(continued)*

CDC Classification

The Centers for Disease Control and Prevention (CDC) uses four groups to characterize stages of HIV disease, with the fourth group consisting of five subgroups. Compared to the Walter Reed system, the CDC system relies more heavily on the patient's condition as its underlying basis.

Class	Description
Group I Acute HIV infection	An individual with HIV infection may experience an acute clinical syndrome approximately 3 to 6 weeks after primary infection. The syndrome has been likened to acute infectious mononucleosis.
Group II Asymptomatic HIV infection	This period marks the length of time from initial infection to the development of clinical disease. The average amount of time this period lasts is 10 years.
Group III Persistent generalized lymphadenopathy	Enlarged lymph nodes in two or more extrainguinal sites without an obvious cause is often the earliest symptom of HIV infection after primary infection.
Group IV Other diseases	Here, the patient develops signs and symptoms of disease other than or in addition to lymphadenopathy:
Group IV-A Constitutional disease	During this stage, the patient may experience fever, diarrhea lasting more than 1 month, and weight loss of 10% of baseline body weight.
Group IV-B Neurologic disease	This class is marked by development of neurologic disorders such as dementia, peripheral neuropathy, and myelopathy.

Classifying HIV disease (continued)

CDC Classification (continued)

Class	Description
Group IV-C Secondary infectious disease	This class is marked by a CD4+ cell count less than 200/µl and the presence of one or more opportunistic infections.
Group IV-D Secondary neoplasms	This class is marked by secondary malignancies, such as invasive cervical carcinoma and Kaposi's sarcoma.
Group IV-E Other conditions	This stage marks development of other conditions related to HIV infection or immunodeficiency and, possibly, coexisting illness indicating immune defect.

Medical history

Also, ask about the patient's medical history, such as:
• whether similar symptoms have occurred in the past
• doctor's visits, diagnoses, and treatments
• past hospitalizations
• prescriptions, including experimental, herbal, and over-the-counter medications
• history of meningitis or brain tumor
• drug and alcohol use

• food, drug, or other allergies.

Skin

Review with the patient possible skin changes, such as the appearance of:
• dermatitis
• dryness
• folliculitis
• local infections or inflammation
• molluscum contagiosum (a viral infection of the skin)
• poor skin turgor
• rash or other lesions
• unusual, unexplained lesions.

Head and neck

Ask the patient about signs and symptoms in his head and neck, such as the occurrence of:
• hair loss
• headaches
• neck stiffness
• oral thrush
• sinusitis
• swollen lymph nodes
• tinnitus
• visual disturbances.

Cardiopulmonary system

Check with the patient about cardiopulmonary symptoms he may be experiencing, such as:

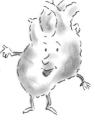

- chest pain
- cyanosis
- dyspnea or other respiratory problems
- hemoptysis
- palpitations or irregular pulse
- pedal edema
- pneumonia
- sputum production.

GI system

Ask the patient about gastrointestinal signs and symptoms, such as:

- abdominal pain
- anorexia
- diarrhea
- esophageal pain or dysphagia
- gastric reflux or dyspepsia
- history of pancreatitis or hepatitis
- nausea and vomiting
- rectal bleeding or lesions
- weight loss.

Neurologic system

Ask the patient about neurologic disturbances, such as:

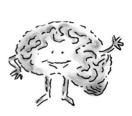

- changes in level of consciousness
- incontinence
- lack of concentration or loss of memory
- motor, sensory, or gait disturbances
- paralysis or weakness in extremities
- seizures
- symptoms of cranial nerve abnormalities
- tingling or pain in fingers or toes.

Hematologic system

Ask the patient if he has been told he has, or currently has symptoms of, the following:

- anemia
- leukopenia (low white blood cell count)
- thrombocytopenia
- tendency to bruise easily
- swollen lymph nodes.

Endocrine system

Ask the patient about endocrine symptoms, such as:

- hypoglycemia (fatigue, restlessness, irritability)
- hyperglycemia (excessive thirst, urination, or eating; unexplained weight loss; fatigue)
- hyponatremia (headache, nausea, abdominal cramps, muscle weakness).

Genitourinary system

Determine whether the patient has signs and symptoms of genitourinary problems. Those signs and symptoms include:

- dysuria
- generalized edema
- oliguria
- penile or vaginal lesions
- proctitis
- sexually transmitted diseases.

Family and social history

Review the patient's family and social history, including:

- general health of his blood relatives, spouse or companion, and sexual partners
- his occupation
- his cohabitants
- his home environment.

Sexual history

Tactfully ask the patient about his sexual history, including:

- current sexual activity
- number and gender of partners

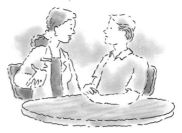

I realize talking about sex can be uncomfortable but I need to ask these questions to obtain an accurate health history.

- condom use
- use of safer sex practices.

Nutritional assessment

A baseline nutritional assessment should include:
- body mass index
- present height and weight
- triceps skinfold measurement
- weight 6 and 12 months ago.
  Blood tests for a nutritional assessment should include:
- albumin
- blood urea nitrogen and creatinine
- cholesterol
- hemoglobin
- liver enzymes
- total iron-binding capacity
- triglyceride levels.

Performing a physical assessment

When performing a physical assessment for a patient who has (or may have) AIDS, remember the general principles of look, listen, and feel. Be sensitive to the patient's privacy and promote a comfortable atmosphere.

Inspection

Perform an inspection for:
- alopecia
- lymphadenopathy
- oral lesions or thrush
- unexplained bruising or poor skin turgor.

  Inspect the patient with Kaposi's sarcoma for:
- changes in gait or locomotion
- hemoptysis
- local inflammation
- rash
- rectal lesions
- urethral discharge.

Palpation

Perform palpation for:
- abdominal pain
- lymphadenopathy
- neck stiffness
- pedal edema
- retro-orbital pain
- sinus pain.

Percussion

Percuss for:
- consolidation in lung fields
- retro-orbital pain
- sinus pain.

Auscultation

Auscultate for:
- adventitious lung sounds
- arrhythmia
- hyperactive peristalsis.

Diagnostic tests

The CDC recommends testing for HIV 3 months after a possible exposure, the approximate length of time before antibodies can be detected in the blood. Not uncommonly, however, an infected patient can test negative for as long as 6 months after exposure. In rare instances, a patient may test negative for as long as 35 months after exposure.

ELISA

The most common test used to detect HIV antibodies is the enzyme-linked immunosorbent assay (ELISA). In the ELISA, the patient's serum sample is incubated with live HIV. If HIV antibodies are present in the blood, the antibodies will react with the test solution.

Here we go again

The ELISA can produce positive results that are actually false, so any positive result of a first ELISA must be validated by a second.

An ELISA can also provide false-negative results if HIV-2 infection is present. (See *Let's confirm it,* page 54.)

Other tests

Other diagnostic tests for HIV measure the severity of the patient's immunosuppression and provide a baseline for comparison. They include:

- anergy testing
- CD4+ and CD8+ cell counts
- complete blood count
- erythrocyte sedimentation rate
- HIV culture
- neopterin levels
- p24 antigen
- serum beta microglobulin
- viral load for HIV. (See *Testing neonates for HIV,* page 55, and *Confidential vs. anonymous testing,* page 56.)

Because of the risk of opportunistic infection, tests may be given to check for a number of infectious

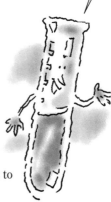

In the ELISA, the patient's serum sample is incubated with live HIV.

Let's confirm it

A Western blot assay must be performed to confirm positive enzyme-linked immunosorbent assay (ELISA) results. The Western blot assay, a more definitive test, can identify specific HIV antibodies and is considered the confirming test for HIV infection.

Positive test results on the ELISA and the Western blot assay mean the patient has been exposed to HIV and has developed antibodies to it. The test itself doesn't necessarily mean the patient has AIDS.

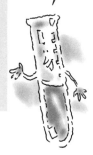

A positive result requires a second test.

diseases, including:
- cytomegalovirus
- hepatitis B
- histoplasmosis
- syphilis
- toxoplasmosis
- tuberculosis.

Put it to the p24 antigen test

The p24 antigen test can detect HIV antigens (HIV p24 core protein) as early as 2 weeks after infection. Studies have indicated a faster progression to AIDS in patients with HIV antigen levels. High levels of anti-

Testing neonates for HIV

Antibody tests in neonates may be unreliable because maternal antibodies still present in the neonate's bloodstream may last up to 10 months, creating a false-positive result. The recommended protocol for neonate testing involves an initial screening with an enzyme-linked immunosorbent assay (ELISA). If positive, another ELISA is performed on the same sample.

Confirming the diagnosis

If both tests are positive, the findings are confirmed by a Western blot assay or, if the child is under age 15 months, an immunofluorescence assay.

Other tests performed to confirm a positive ELISA in children under age 15 months include increased levels of serum immunoglobulins, decreased lymphocyte count or $CD8^+$ count, or a decrease in the helper T-cell to suppressor T-cell ratio. A positive HIV serum antigen or HIV culture also helps to confirm a positive ELISA.

gens indicate that the virus is actively replicating.

Waiting for the results

An HIV culture detects live HIV but can take up to 4 weeks to produce results. The test measures the amount of reverse transcriptase activity. Reverse transcriptase is responsible for protein synthesis, which allows for growth of the virus.

Advice from the experts

Confidential vs. anonymous testing

Does confidential testing mean no one else will know the results of the HIV testing? No. It's important to understand that if an HIV test is paid for by an employer or insurance company, the company will learn the results.

No one else will know

Anonymous testing, on the other hand, provides no documented evidence of HIV status. Normally those receiving an anonymous test are given a code name or number to which the results are matched. The test results aren't traceable. No written documentation of the results is available to a third party.

Rules and recommendations

Keep these facts in mind about HIV testing:

• No one can perform an HIV test without written permission.

• Tell the patient to read all documents carefully, especially insurance documents, before signing blanket waivers for release of medical records or giving permission for laboratory work.

• Remember that, to provide informed consent, a patient must be adequately counseled before signing a consent form for an HIV test.

What is there to say about a T-cell assay?

Also known as an immune profile, a T-cell assay measures the number of T cells in the bloodstream. The extent of T-cell reduction — both helper T cells and suppressor T cells — usually parallels the disease stage.

Helper T cells stimulate B cells to mature into plasma cells, which synthesize and secrete immunoglobulins, or proteins with antibody activities. Suppressor T cells reduce the body's humoral (immunoglobulin-mediated) response. With HIV infection, the number of helper T cells usually decreases while the number of suppressor T cells increases.

The lowdown on viral load

Viral load measures the number of ribonucleic acid (RNA) strands of HIV in the plasma or serum of an HIV-infected person. Measuring viral load helps make treatment decisions easier at all stages of HIV disease, especially during asymptomatic periods when the helper T-cell count is close to normal. Viral loads usually increase with advanced disease.

As HIV infection progresses, the number of helper T cells dwindles.

What viral load results mean

Researchers continue to fine-tune the use of the viral load test, but as a general guideline, HIV viral loads correlate to the survival rate or the rate of disease progression. Here's a breakdown of what the results mean.

Viral load	Meaning
5,000 or lower	Survival rate of 5 years or greater
10,000 or lower	Low risk of disease progression
10,001 to 100,000	Medium risk of disease progression
Over 100,000	High risk of disease progression

Test results are measured in virus particles per milliliters of blood. Keep in mind that blood carries only about 2% of HIV; the lymph system and other body tissues hold the other 98%.

Viral load tests may also serve as an indicator of successful treatment. If a patient begins a new therapy and viral loads decrease at least by half of the previous result, then the new therapy is considered effective. (See *What viral load results mean.*)

Absence of a reaction

Anergy testing can identify people with inadequate immune systems. Anergy is the absence of a reaction to a known reactant. Anergy testing typically consists of skin tests for mumps, *Candida,* and tuberculosis.

A person with a strong immune system will have a positive reaction to the mumps and *Candida* and a negative reaction to tuberculosis skin tests. People exposed to tuberculosis, who have active tuberculosis, and who have received bacille Calmette-Guérin immunizations will also have a positive reaction to tuberculosis skin tests.

Patients with HIV infection and immune system deficits will often show anergy. Absence of a reaction during anergy testing in the presence of clinical symptoms of decreased immunity may indicate the need for further tests. If a patient's immune system is severely depleted, anergy testing may not be sufficient. Further tests for tuberculosis may be necessary and typically consist of chest X-rays, sputum cultures, and bronchoscopy.

Quick quiz

1. The average length of the latent period for HIV infection in an adult is:

    A.   2 years.

    B.   5 years.

    C.   10 years.

Answer: C. HIV has a long incubation period. In adults, the average latent period is 10 years.

2. An HIV test drawn yesterday reveals the patient's HIV status from:

    A.   1 week ago.

    B.   3 months ago.

    C.   9 months ago.

Answer: B. Because of the window period for seroconversion, an HIV test generally reveals the person's HIV status as of 3 months ago.

3. HIV diagnosis in an adult is confirmed by:

    A.   ELISA.

    B.   p24 antigen test.

    C.   Western blot assay.

Answer: C. The Western blot assay is considered the confirming test; the ELISA is the screening test.

4. Children under age 15 months are more difficult to test accurately for HIV because:

    A. large blood specimens are difficult to obtain.

    B. the child's body hasn't produced HIV antibodies yet.

    C. maternal antibodies are still present and may create a false-positive result.

Answer: C. Maternal antibodies still present in the infant's bloodstream may provide a false-positive result to HIV testing.

5. For the majority of HIV-infected people, the window period (the period of infection without antibodies) lasts:

    A. 10 years.

    B. 6 months.

    C. less than 3 months.

Answer: C. For the majority of patients who are infected with HIV, the window period lasts less than 3 months.

6. In its early stages, HIV infection tends to produce:

    A.   specific and easily recognizable changes in the body

    B.   subtle and nonspecific changes in the body

    C.   complex and wide-ranging infections and diseases.

Answer: B. In its early stages, HIV infection tends to produce subtle and nonspecific changes in the body.

Scoring

☆☆☆   If you answered all six questions correctly, fabulous! The window period for your learning is narrow indeed!

  ☆☆   If you answered three or more questions correctly, terrific! You've reduced your transmission of errors.

    ☆   If you answered fewer than three questions correctly, don't worry. Follow-up testing is important in any field.

4

Treating patients with AIDS

> ### Key facts
> ◆ Nucleoside analogue reverse transcriptase inhibitors slow replication of HIV by blocking the reverse transcriptase enzyme.
> ◆ Non-nucleoside reverse transcriptase inhibitors also slow replication of HIV by blocking the reverse transcriptase enzyme.
> ◆ Protease inhibitors inhibit the activity of HIV protease, an enzyme essential for replication in chronically infected cells.
> ◆ Combination therapy, called highly active antiretroviral therapy (HAART), is the standard treatment for HIV infection.
> ◆ Complementary therapies have become an integral part of HIV-AIDS treatment.

Drugs

Drugs used to treat HIV and AIDS work in one of three ways:

 slowing replication of the virus

 suppressing, preventing, or stopping

the recurrence of opportunistic infections

 boosting the immune system.

Three families

Drugs to treat AIDS generally fall into three families, categorized by how they affect HIV. They are:
• nucleoside analogue reverse transcriptase inhibitors (NARTIs)
• non-nucleoside reverse transcriptase inhibitors (NNRTIs)
• protease inhibitors (PIs). (See *AIDS medications*.)

Fusion inhibitors are a fourth class under development. These drugs prevent HIV from entering healthy cells.

(Text continues on page 75.)

Some drugs prevent me from replicating quickly...

...while others boost the immune system.

AIDS medications

NARTIs

Nucleoside analogue reverse transcriptase inhibitors (NARTIs) slow the replication of HIV by blocking the reverse transcriptase enzyme. This enzyme, present in HIV, is necessary for the virus to enter a cell and integrate into the cell's genetic material. Without reverse transcriptase, the HIV virus doesn't replicate. Drugs in this group include abacavir, didanosine, lamivudine, lamivudine-zidovudine, stavudine, zalcitabine, and zidovudine.

abacavir (1592U89)
Trade name: Ziagen

Adverse reactions
Major: nausea, vomiting, diarrhea, anorexia, insomnia, headache, and abnormal liver function

Special considerations
• Monitor for liver dysfunction.
• Fever, rash, vomiting, diarrhea, or abdominal pain may signal the beginning of a hypersensitivity reaction. The patient should seek medical attention immediately and shouldn't attempt to take the drug again.
• Abacavir is a component of combination therapy with zidovudine and lamivudine.

didanosine (ddI)
Trade name: Videx

Adverse reactions
• Major: peripheral neuropathy, pancreatitis, anxiety, headache, insomnia, restlessness, dry mouth, nervousness, rash, seizures, nausea, vomiting, and thrombocytopenia
• Unusual: possible retinal depigmentation in children

(continued)

AIDS medications *(continued)*

Special considerations
- Give on an empty stomach 1 hour before or 2 hours after meals.
- Chew tablets thoroughly, with at least 1oz of water.
- If taking powder, dissolve completely in 4 oz of nonacidic beverage.
- Don't administer with acidic beverages (such as citrus juices).
- Don't give within 2 hours of dapsone or ketoconazole because of buffering effect of didanosine on gastric pH.
- May increase absorption of tetracycline and fluoroquinolones.
- Concurrent use of antacids may increase diarrhea or constipation.
- Use cautiously in those with renal or liver impairment.
- Children undergoing therapy require a dilated eye examination every 6 months.
- Didanosine is a component of combination therapy.

lamivudine (3TC)
Trade name: Epivir

Adverse reactions
Major: pancreatitis, alopecia, peripheral neuropathy, fatigue, weakness, fever, chills, rash, nausea, headache, diarrhea, cough, abdominal cramps, and dyspepsia

Special considerations
- Tell the patient to avoid alcohol.
- Monitor complete blood count (CBC), platelet count, and liver function.
- Assess the patient for symptoms of pancreatitis.
- Trimethoprim with sulfamethoxazole may increase absorption of lamivudine.
- Lamivudine is a component of combination therapy.

lamivudine-zidovudine
Trade name: Combivir

AIDS medications *(continued)*

Adverse reactions

Major: anemia, nausea, headache, fatigue, muscle pain, vomiting, insomnia, neutropenia (commonly indicated by sore throat with fever and chills), bone marrow depression, pancreatitis, peripheral neuropathy, weakness, rash, diarrhea, and cough

Special considerations

• Monitor CBC.
• Monitor patients for signs of lactic acidosis and hepatotoxicity.
• Monitor patient's fine motor skills and peripheral sensation for peripheral neuropathy.
• Combination may be given with or without food.
• Immediately report symptoms of neutropenia, anemia, or pancreatitis (such as fever, sore throat, light-headedness, pale skin, weakness, or abdominal pain).
• Lamivudine-zidovudine is a combination therapy that facilitates longer use of other drugs.

stavudine (d4T)

Trade name: Zerit

Adverse reactions

Major: peripheral neuropathy, headache, diarrhea, fever, chills, nausea, vomiting, lack of energy, insomnia, anxiety, dizziness, and anorexia

Special considerations

• The drug may be taken without regard to meals.
• Advise against using alcohol when taking this drug.
• Monitor the patient's liver function.
• Use cautiously in patients with renal impairment or history of peripheral neuropathy. Adjust dose or discontinue use in the event of peripheral neuropathy.
• Tell the patient to report symptoms of peripheral neuropathy (pain, burning, aching,

(continued)

AIDS medications *(continued)*

weakness, or pins and needles in the extremities) immediately.
• Stavudine is a component of combination therapy.

zalcitabine (dideoxycytidine, ddC)
Trade name: HIVID

Adverse reactions
• Major: peripheral neuropathy, mouth ulcers, oral lesions, abdominal pain, nausea, vomiting, rash, GI intolerance, pruritus, muscle pain, difficulty swallowing, and arthralgia
• Additional: headache, fatigue, seizures, heart failure, neutropenia, leukopenia, fever, thrombocytopenia, and erythematous, maculopapular, or follicular rash

Special considerations
• Best taken on an empty stomach.
• Advise the patient to swallow capsules whole, with plenty of water.
• Use cautiously with drugs that may cause peripheral neuropathy or renal toxicity.
• Concurrent use of pentamidine may lead to pancreatitis. Concurrent use of cimetidine decreases elimination of zalcitabine.

zidovudine (ZDV, azidothymidine, AZT)
Trade name: Retrovir

Adverse reactions
• Major: anemia, nausea, headache, fatigue, muscle pain, vomiting, insomnia, neutropenia (commonly indicated by sore throat with fever and chills), bone marrow depression, confusion, mental changes, seizures, dizziness, abdominal pain, diarrhea, and lethargy
• Unusual: blue-brown bands on fingernails

AIDS medications *(continued)*

Special considerations
- Effect of taking medication with food is unknown.
- Protect pills from light.
- Monitor CBC and renal and liver function every 2 weeks.
- Use cautiously with other nephrotoxic or myelotoxic agents.
- Zidovudine is used as prophylaxis for vertical transmission (for example, mother to newborn) and as a component of combination therapy.

NNRTIs

Non-nucleoside reverse transcriptase inhibitor (NNRTI) drugs inhibit replication of HIV by blocking the reverse transcriptase enzyme. NNRTIs cause changes in the reverse transcriptase enzyme that render it inactive. Drugs in this group include delavirdine, efavirenz, and nevirapine.

delavirdine
Trade name: Rescriptor

Adverse reactions
Major: rash, arthralgia, change in dreams, nausea, diarrhea, fatigue, neutropenia, pancytopenia, thrombocytopenia, Stevens-Johnson syndrome, and elevated liver enzymes

Special considerations
- Monitor liver function.
- Rash usually occurs within the first 3 weeks.
- Resistance develops rapidly, so always use delavirdine in combination therapy.

(continued)

AIDS medications *(continued)*

efavirenz (DMP-266)
Trade name: Sustiva

Adverse reactions
Major: dizziness, nightmares, headache, light-headedness, and rash

Special considerations
- Don't administer this drug to a pregnant woman as it may cause birth defects.
- Efavirenz is used in combination therapy with zidovudine and indinavir.

nevirapine
Trade name: Viramune

Adverse reactions
Major: oral lesions, abnormal liver function, hepatitis, headache, rash, fever, nausea, neutropenia, Stevens-Johnson syndrome, numbness, and muscle pain

Special considerations
- Monitor liver function.
- Nevirapine can decrease plasma concentrations of protease inhibitors or oral contraceptives and shouldn't be administered concurrently.
- Monitor for blistering, oral lesions, conjunctivitis, myalgia, arthralgia, or general malaise.
- Be alert for rash, especially rash with fever. Most rashes occur within 6 weeks. Report rash to primary care provider.
- Nevirapine is a component of combination therapy.

PIs

Protease inhibitors (PIs) inhibit the activity of HIV protease, an enzyme essential for replication in chronically infected cells. Inhibiting HIV protease leaves viral particles

AIDS medications *(continued)*

noninfectious. In general, PIs are associated with increased blood glucose and diabetes. Drugs in this group include indinavir, ritonavir, and saquinavir.

indinavir
Trade name: Crixivan

Adverse reactions
Major: kidney stones, altered taste, elevated blood glucose, triglycerides, and cholesterol; possible fat accumulation and development of buffalo hump

Special considerations
- Must be given 1 hour before or after didanosine.
- The patient must drink at least $1\frac{1}{2}$ qt (1.5 L) of water per day, to reduce risk of nephrolithiasis.
- Tell the patient not to take indinavir with citrus juice.
- Use cautiously with renal or hepatic insufficiency. Notify primary care provider of signs of nephrolithiasis, such as flank pain and hematuria.
- Indinavir is moisture-sensitive; keep it in the original container with desiccants to prevent moisture from accumulating.
- Indinavir is best taken with a light, low-fat, low-protein meal.
- Indinavir is used as part of combination therapy.

nelfinavir
Trade name: Viracept

Adverse reactions
Major: diarrhea, elevated blood glucose, seizures, depression, leukopenia, thrombocytopenia, hepatitis, fat accumulation, and development of buffalo hump

Special considerations
- Consider giving loperamide for diarrhea.

(continued)

AIDS medications *(continued)*

• Administer with meal or light snack, to increase bioavailability.
• Don't administer this drug with acidic foods or juices, as it will produce a bitter taste.
• Nelfinavir is used as part of combination therapy.

---

ritonavir

Trade name: Norvir

Adverse reactions

Major: nausea; vomiting; diarrhea; abdominal pain; taste alterations; dizziness; headache; leukopenia, thrombocytopenia; tingling or numbness around hands, feet, or lips; fatigue; weakness; possible elevated blood glucose, triglycerides, cholesterol, and liver enzymes; and buffalo hump

Special considerations

• Refrigerate capsules; keep oral solution at room temperature and protect it from light.
• Administer capsules with food, oral solution without food.
• Advise the patient to disguise the taste with ice or strong flavors, such as chocolate milk, Ensure, or Advera (none of which will affect bioavailability).
• Use cautiously with hepatic insufficiency.
• Starting ritonavir alone, then adding nucleosides within 2 weeks may improve GI tolerance.
• Tobacco decreases serum levels.
• Monitor blood glucose, triglyceride, cholesterol, and liver function levels.
• Be aware that ritonavir interacts with drugs from many different classes — for example, nicotine, alphazolam, theophylline, rifampin, and propoxyphene.
• Ritonavir is a component of combination therapy.

AIDS medications (continued)

saquinavir
Trade names: Invirase, Fortovase

Adverse reactions
• Major: nausea; diarrhea; oral lesions; abdominal pain; elevated blood glucose, triglyceride, and cholesterol levels; and possible photosensitivity
• Unusual: development of a buffalo hump or redistribution of fat often called the "protease paunch"

Special considerations
• Saquinavir is compounded with lactose; if the patient is lactose intolerant, advise him to take lactose-intolerance tablets (Lactaid) before taking the drug.
• Saquinavir should be taken at mealtime.
• Monitor CBC and blood glucose, cholesterol, triglyceride, uric acid, and electrolyte levels.
• Be aware that rifabutin and rifampin reduce saquinavir levels.
• Interaction with astemizole or cisapride many cause serious adverse reactions.
• Saquinavir is a component of combination therapy.

Drugs under investigation

Unlike other drug classifications, experimental drugs may each have very different effects on the body. What unifies this group is that the drugs are all relatively new. Given the fact that traditional medications have yet to provide a cure for HIV, these drugs are worthy of investigation. Common experimental drugs include adefovir, ABT-378, amprenavir (141W94), and hydroxyurea.

(continued)

AIDS medications *(continued)*

adefovir

Trade name: Preveon

Adverse reactions

Major: nausea, vomiting, anorexia, and elevated liver enzymes

Special considerations
• Advise the patient to take L-carnitine supplements (available over-the-counter) to help break down proteins and fats.
• Adefovir is used as part of combination therapy.

ABT-378

Trade name: unnamed

Adverse reactions

Major: diarrhea, headache, and weakness

Special considerations
• Remind the patient that this drug is still under investigation for use in HIV and AIDS therapy.
• ABT-378 is a new second-generation protease inhibitor.

amprenavir (141W94)

Trade name: Agenerase

Adverse reactions

Major: diarrhea, headache, nausea, and abdominal pain

Special considerations
• Advise the patient to take this drug with food.
• Remind him that this drug is still under investigation for HIV and AIDS therapy.
• Amprenavir is a PI under investigation for use when other therapies fail.

AIDS medications (continued)

hydroxyurea
Trade name: Hydrea

Adverse reactions

Major: bone marrow depression; leukopenia; anemia, which requires transfusions; renal toxicity, which requires laboratory monitoring; and hallucinations, which increase when renal function decreases

Special considerations
- Hydroxyurea is usually taken with didanosine or didanosine and stavudine. These combinations save PIs and NNRTIs for later use if therapy is less than successful.
- Currently, there is no documented resistance to this drug and it costs less than others. However, it isn't recommended for monotherapy.
- Administer cautiously with zidovudine.
- Remind the patient that this drug is still under investigation for HIV and AIDS therapy.
- Because it interrupts the cell cycle, hydroxyurea is also used as a treatment for cancer and sickle cell anemia.

Combination therapy

Combination therapy for HIV-AIDS, often called highly active antiretroviral therapy (HAART), is the recommended treatment for HIV infection. This therapy usually combines a PI with a NARTI, a NNRTI, or both in order to:
- reduce mutation

- decrease resistance to therapy
- render HIV infection a chronic illness, rather than a deadly illness. (See *The Heart of HAART.*)

Up to 90%

Research has shown that HAART can reduce opportunistic infections by up to 90%. If tolerated, HAART can improve the overall health and quality of life for many patients. Unfortunately, these drugs have significant adverse effects, including a change in lipid metabolism that results in redistribution of body fat and elevated cholesterol counts.

Drug resistance is the biggest threat to the long-term use of combination therapy. HIV develops resistance to antiviral drugs in roughly the same way bacteria become resistant to antibiotics, but HIV develops resistance at a much more rapid rate.

Drug resistance testing is becoming more accurate. Increased accuracy helps clinicians decide which components of a patient's regimen to change.

The heart of HAART

Highly active antiretroviral therapy (HAART) usually consists of protease inhibitors (PIs) combined with nucleoside analogue reverse transcriptase inhibitors (NARTIs) or non-nucleoside reverse transcriptase inhibitors (NNRTIs) or both.

PIs	NARTIs	NNRTIs
indinavir	abacavir	delavirdine
nelfinavir	adefovir	efavirenz
ritonavir	didanosine	nevirapine
saquinavir	lamivudine	
	stavudine	
	zalcitabine	
	zidovudine	

When to treat HIV

Many experts support the treatment of acute primary HIV infections, regardless of the patient's CD4+ or viral load levels or whether the patient is experiencing symptoms. Other primary care providers are more conservative and wait until CD4+ levels drop below 500, viral loads increase over 10,000, or the patient develops symptoms. The decision when to start any treatment should be made in consultation with the patient's primary care provider, based on the most current research findings. The patient's right to informed consent must be respected in all treatment decisions.

Complementary therapy

Complementary therapy has become integral to treatment of HIV and AIDS. Many people with HIV infection believe that such treatments as special diets, Chinese herbs, and vitamin preparations

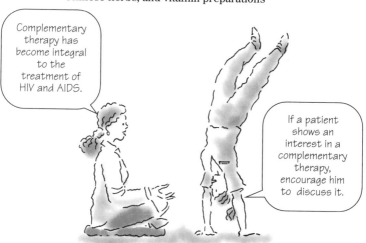

Complementary therapy has become integral to the treatment of HIV and AIDS.

If a patient shows an interest in a complementary therapy, encourage him to discuss it.

will help control HIV infection. The effectiveness of these treatments hasn't been tested in clinical trials.

Don't keep it a secret

Studies indicate that many patients use a complementary therapy without informing their primary care provider because they fear a negative response. If a patient shows an interest in a complementary therapy, encourage him to discuss it.

Common complements

Most standard medications treat HIV directly, attacking the pathogens in the body. By contrast, complementary therapies seek to treat the individual holistically, building up the person's strength (including the immune system).

Examples of common complementary therapies for HIV-AIDS include:

- acupuncture
- aromatherapy
- biofeedback
- herbal medicine
- meditation
- nutrition
- *qi gong*
- yoga.

Acupuncture

Acupuncture, which comes from traditional Chinese medicine, receives more federal funding than any other complementary therapy in the United States. According to Chinese medicine, sickness results from an imbalance in the body's energy flow (*Qi*, pronounced "chee"). Using thin needles, inserted into specific "acupoints" on the skin, acupuncture helps the body regain balance (homeostasis).

Proponents of acupuncture report many benefits. Patients generally feel better, physically and emotionally, when receiving regular treatment. They also report that acupuncture alleviates many adverse reactions to AIDS medications. Proponents claim that, if treatment begins early enough, acupuncture may prevent HIV from causing extensive damage.

Aromatherapy

Aromas, whether we notice them or not, affect moods and thought patterns. Based on this idea, aromatherapy uses essential plant oils to create pleasant sensations and promote relaxation. This type of therapy may be beneficial to an AIDS patient suffering from depression or lethargy.

Biofeedback

Biofeedback therapy uses electronic instruments to display blood pressure, heart rate, respiratory rate, and temperature. The feedback allows a patient to become aware of these bodily functions. When a person becomes aware of these functions, he can bring them under conscious control (with practice). Biofeedback is especially useful for relieving symptoms of stress and anxiety.

Herbal medicine

Ask your patient if he's taking any herbal remedies. If so, ask how he learned about these remedies and if he's under the care of an herbalist. Discuss possible benefits and risks with the patient, including the risk of interactions with prescribed drugs. (For more about herbs used to treat HIV, see *Herbal remedies,* pages 82 to 85.)

Meditation

Meditation promotes relaxation. It is the practice of being mindful or aware. One central feature of meditation is the focus

(Text continues on page 86.)

Herbal remedies

Attitudes toward herbal remedies are changing dramatically. With the advent of modern medicine, herbal remedies lost credibility as effective treatment for most illnesses. Now, however, pharmacies, health food stores, and supermarkets devote entire shelves to herbal remedies. In fact, herbal agents are the top-selling over-the-counter "medications" in the United States.

Debate continues among health care professionals regarding the efficacy of herbal medicine. The Food and Drug Administration (FDA) doesn't regulate use or manufacture of most herbal agents.

Below are ten herbal agents that your HIV or AIDS patient may be taking. Remember that, for all of the following agents, few clinical studies involving humans have been performed.

Cat's-claw

Also known by the trade names Cat's Claw Inner Bark Extract and Vegicaps, cat's-claw's active components are extracted from the roots, stem bark, and leaves of *Uncaria tomentosa*, a woody vine native to the Amazon region.

Four cat's-claw alkaloids have shown immunostimulating properties in vitro. Their effects include enhanced helper T-cell function.

A patient taking cat's-claw runs the risk of hypotension, so tell the patient to avoid taking antihypertensives with cat's-claw. The patient should also watch for any bleeding. More research is necessary to determine the efficacy and safety of cat's claw.

Chaparral

Chaparral's active components are extracted from the leaves of *Larrea tridentata*, a desert evergreen shrub native to the southwestern United States and Mexico.

Herbal remedies *(continued)*

The biological activity of chaparral is attributed to NDGA, a lipoxygenase inhibitor used as a food additive. NDGA reportedly interrupts the life cycle of HIV.

Possible adverse reactions include contact dermatitis, renal cell carcinoma, and renal cystic disease as well as hepatotoxicity, according to numerous reports. The FDA has removed this herb from its "generally recognized as safe" list. No drug interactions have been reported.

Daffodil

Active components of daffodil are derived from the powders or extracts of the flower *Narcissus pseudonarcissus*, commonly found in Europe and the United States.

NPA, the lectin found in daffodil bulbs, is used in biochemical research because of its ability to bind with glycoconjugates on viruses, including HIV-1 and HIV-2.

Daffodil flowers and bulbs are poisonous. Even ingestion of small quantities can lead to rapid death, so warn your patient against eating any part of this plant. When taken properly as an alternative medicine, possible adverse reactions include contact dermatitis, hypersalivation, miosis, nausea, vomiting, and respiratory and cardiovascular collapse. Although research is in progress, this herb isn't currently recommended for internal use. No drug interactions have been reported.

Iceland moss

A lichen that grows in the Northern hemisphere, Iceland moss, or *Cetraria islandica,* is common in the mountains and heathlands of Iceland.

In vitro evidence has shown that protolichesterinic acid from Iceland moss inhibits activity of HIV-1 reverse transcriptase. In Europe, extracts from Iceland moss have been used for treatment of throat irritation and coughs, tuberculosis, asthma, and GI disorders. Adverse reactions associated with large doses or prolonged use include GI irritation and liver toxicity. Signs of toxicity include abdominal pain, diarrhea, nausea, vomiting, and bleeding as well as changes in color of urine, stool, or skin. No drug interactions have been reported.

(continued)

Herbal remedies (continued)

Marigold

Active components of marigold are extracted from the small yellow-orange flower heads of *Calendula officinalis*. Marigold is native to southern Europe and the eastern Mediterranean; it also grows in many parts of the United States and Canada.

Marigold extract appears to have antiviral properties that fight HIV-1. Allergic reactions have been reported with other members of the marigold family. No drug interactions have been reported.

Schisandra

Also called Sheng-mai-san, active components of *Schisandra chinesis* are extracted from the fruit, stems, and kernel by using ethanol. The plant is native to China, Russia, and Korea.

In vitro, a component of schisandra has been found to inhibit reverse transcriptase. In rare cases, central nervous system (CNS) depression has been reported as an adverse reaction. Although no drug interactions have been reported, schisandra may interfere with the liver's ability to eliminate other drugs.

Self-heal

Self-heal is an herbal remedy derived from *Prunella vulgaris*, commonly found in fields, grassy areas, and woods of North America, Asia, and Europe.

Prunellin, an aqueous extract of the herb, has shown antiviral activity against HIV-1 in vitro. Aqueous extracts have the most antiviral activity. This remedy appears promising, but needs more research to determine efficacy and safety.

Take special precautions when caring for a patient taking prunellin. Monitor liver function periodically. Because of toxicity, large doses should be avoided. Commercial sources have been found to be contaminated with other herbs. More research is needed to determine efficacy and safety. No adverse reactions or drug interactions have been reported.

Herbal remedies *(continued)*

Skullcap

This herbal remedy is made from the leaves and roots of the plants *Scutellaria lateriflolia* and *S. baicalensis*, which are prepared as hot water or methanolic extracts. The plants are native to temperate regions of North America.

Baicalin, an extract of skullcap, reportedly inhibits HIV-1 infection and HIV-1 replication in human peripheral blood cells.

Reported adverse reactions include hepatotoxicity, arrhythmias, confusion, giddiness, seizures, stupor, and twitching. The patient shouldn't take skullcap with disulfiram or immunosuppressive agents.

Spirulina

Spirulina is an algae that thrives in the highly alkaline waters of subtropical and tropical areas. Calcium spirulan, a sulfated polysaccharide compound formulated from the algae's lipid content, has shown a high selectivity index for inhibiting the replication of HIV-1 and other viruses.

Spirulina can contain significant amounts of mercury and other metals. It may contain radioactive divalent and trivalent metallic ions, depending on where it's manufactured. No adverse reactions or drug interactions have been reported.

Thuja

Active components of thuja are obtained from the needles and young twigs of *Thuja occidentalis*, which is an evergreen conifer native to eastern North America.

Thuja inhibits HIV-1 antigens and HIV-2 specific reverse transcriptase. It can induce a subset of T cells.

Adverse reactions may include asthma, CNS stimulation, flatulence, seizures, stomach irritation, and uterine stimulation that may lead to spontaneous abortion. If the patient is taking an anticonvulsant (which raises the seizure threshold), thuja may counteract that effect (lowering the seizure threshold). Adjust anticonvulsant dosage as needed. Also, tell your patient to avoid caffeine and other stimulants because of an additive effect.

on breathing. The patient should let the mind wander, noticing thoughts without clinging to them, then bring attention back to the breath. Practicing meditation for even a few minutes every day can help AIDS patients gain peace of mind.

Nutrition

Good nutrition is an essential part of any patient's therapy. The patient should eat a diet high in protein and calories to combat weight loss that accompanies AIDS. Drinking water should be purified (filtered, bottled, or boiled) to prevent exposure to microbes. Consider referring the patient to a professional nutritionist.

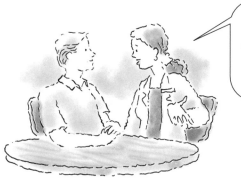

Feel free to discuss any complementary therapies that are of interest to you.

Qi gong and yoga

Qi (mentioned in relation to acupuncture) is the body's life energy. The body needs to move to be healthy. *Qi gong* uses slow-motion, low-impact exercises to improve circulation. Yoga, a similar practice, involves more stretching.

Surgery

In patients with HIV, surgery may be used as a diagnostic procedure, as in bronchoscopy and biopsy. Surgery may also treat secondary manifestations of the immunocompromised state caused by HIV. For example, cancers of the female reproductive tract may be treated with hysterectomy.

Other treatments

When treating HIV and AIDS, also remember to:
• avoid administering live vaccines
• conduct regular, thorough follow-ups.

Hold it

An HIV-positive patient shouldn't receive live virus or bacteria vaccines (measles-mumps-rubella, oral polio vaccine, bacilli Calmette-Guérin, typhoid vaccine). Administer yellow fever vaccine only if the risk of infection exceeds that of adverse effects. Administer other nonliving or nonbacterial vaccines based on the risk of disease and the effectiveness of the vaccine.

Although you should avoid administering many vaccines to HIV patients, the Centers for Disease Control and Prevention recommends that patients receive influenza virus vaccine and *Pneumoniae* (pneumoniae polysaccharide) vaccine.

I'll see you in 3 months

For asymptomatic HIV-positive patients, you should conduct a follow-up visit every 3 to 6 months. It should include:
• history and physical examination every year
• CD4+ and CD8+ counts and ratio every 3 to 4 months and 1 month after any treatment change

- HIV ribonucleic acid plasma levels every 3 to 4 months and 1 month after any treatment change
- complete blood count every year
- chemistry panel every year
- urinalysis every year
- tuberculin skin test every year
- Papanicolaou test every year for women
- Venereal Disease Research Laboratory test every year for sexually active patients
- gonococcal and chlamydial cultures every 6 to 12 months for sexually active patients
- toxoplasmosis serologic test every year.

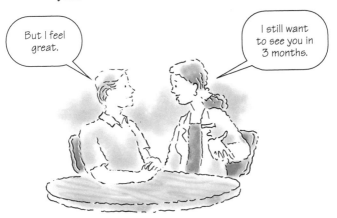

Quick quiz

1. Current drug treatments for HIV infection work by of all the following methods except:

    A. slowing replication of the virus.

    B. killing macrophages.

    C. stopping opportunistic infections.

Answer: B. HIV destroys the immune system's macrophages; killing macrophages only encourages HIV.

2. The drug used for prophylaxis of vertical transmission is:

    A. ritonavir.

    B. zidovudine.

    C. hydroxyurea.

Answer: B. Zidovudine (AZT) stops new strands of HIV DNA from being made by blocking reverse transcriptase.

Scoring

☆☆☆   If you answered both questions correctly, right on! You're developing a resistance to failure.

☆☆   If you answered fewer than two questions correctly, reading the chapter again will act as combination therapy.

5

AIDS-related conditions

Key facts
- ◆ Many complications arise from common pathogens. Complications are made life-threatening by the patient's weakened immune system.
- ◆ Opportunistic infections and malignancies often signal the progression from HIV-positive status to AIDS.
- ◆ AIDS dementia and HIV-AIDS wasting syndrome indicate the later stages of AIDS.

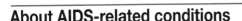

About AIDS-related conditions

Early complications from AIDS usually include:
- development of opportunistic infections
- appearance of malignancies such as Kaposi's sarcoma.

  Later complications from AIDS include:
- AIDS dementia complex
- HIV-AIDS wasting syndrome.

Opportunistic infections

Opportunistic infections occur when pathogens take advantage of the suppressed immune state, especially the T cell's weakened response. These pathogens are often those that the patient encounters in his normal environment but can't fight off because of his weakened immune system.

Resistant and recurring

Opportunistic infections often lead to complicated illnesses that spread quickly through the body. Because of the patient's suppressed immune response, these illnesses tend to resist treatment and recur regularly.

Candidiasis

Candidiasis, a fungal infection commonly known as yeast or thrush, may appear on teeth, gingivae, skin, the vagina, the oropharynx, or the large intestine. When it appears in the vagina, it's often a woman's first AIDS-related infection. Because this type of infection is relatively common, it may not be recognized as a sign of HIV.

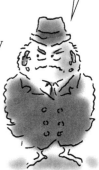

It's true. I depress the immune system, paving the way for infections and tumors.

Look for yellow patches, nail infections...

On cheek and tongue surfaces, look for creamy, curdlike yellow or white patches surrounded by an erythematous base. Also look for painful nail infections or intense pruritus of the vulva and a curdlike discharge. The infection may produce an odor similar to rising bread dough.

Treatment depends on location

The treatment used for candidiasis and its delivery method depends on the loca-

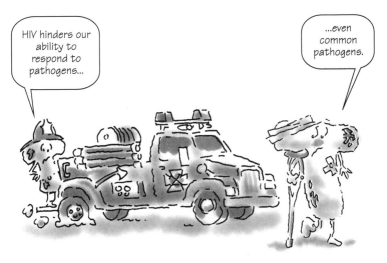

tion of the infection. For thrush, typically use nystatin suspension and clotrimazole troches. For esophagitis, you may use nystatin suspension or pastilles, clotrimazole troches, oral ketoconazole, fluconazole, or itraconazole. Use topical versions of these drugs for cutaneous lesions and suppositories for rectal or vaginal infections. Recurrent or severe vaginal candidiasis may need systemic therapy.

Coccidiosis

The sporozoan infection coccidiosis is caused by the parasites *Isospora hominis* and *I. belli*. These parasites are often ingested and infect the small intestine, resulting in malabsorption and diarrhea. Report outbreaks to local health authorities.

Look for abdominal pain, diarrhea...

Signs and symptoms of coccidiosis include watery, nonbloody diarrhea; cramps or abdominal pain; nausea; anorexia; weight loss; and low grade fever.

Treat with fluconazole, amphotericin B...

Typical drugs include fluconazole, amphotericin B, or itraconazole.

Cryptococcosis

The fungus that causes cryptococcosis often occurs in nature, but normal immune defenses protect against infection. When inhaled, it travels to the lungs. From the lungs, it may disseminate to the central nervous system (CNS) or remain dormant. Symptoms are vague and commonly confused with other opportunistic infections. In some jurisdictions, outbreaks should be reported to local health authorities.

When inhaled, guess where cryptococcosis travels — to yours truly.

Look for cough, fever, chest pain...

Look for the following signs and symptoms of cryptococcosis:
• in the respiratory system — fever, cough, dyspnea, pleuritic chest pain, and hemoptysis
• in the CNS — fever, headache, chills, seizures, stiff neck, vomiting, and altered mentation
• disseminated symptoms — lymphadenopathy, rashes, lesions, myocarditis, optic neuropathy, and rectal abscesses.

Treat with amphotericin B or fluconazole...

Typically, amphotericin B is used to treat inpatients with cryptococcosis; fluconazole is commonly used for outpatients. In some cases, itraconazole may also be used.

Cryptosporidiosis

The protozoan *Cryptosporidium* causes cryptosporidiosis, which usually locates itself in the small intestine. These protozoa travel through fecal-oral contact, oral-anal contact, water, or food contamination. Report outbreaks to local health authorities.

Yeah, I get around. I travel by person-to-person contact, water, or food contamination.

Look for watery diarrhea...

The major symptom in adults is watery diarrhea; also look for abdominal cramping, flatulence, weight loss, anorexia, malaise, fever, and nausea. In children, major symptoms are anorexia and vomiting.

Treatment is supportive

No effective treatment exists to eliminate cryptosporidiosis. Supportive treatment focuses on total parenteral nutrition and fluid replacement. Drug therapy may include spiramycin or quinine and clindamycin.

Cytomegalovirus

A form of herpesvirus, cytomegalovirus (CMV) may result in serious, widespread infection. It's commonly found in the lungs, adrenal glands, eyes, CNS, GI tract, male genitourinary tract, and blood. This virus is spread through blood and body fluids. It can reactivate in an immunocompromised patient.

Be alert for pneumonia, diarrhea, blindness...

For HIV patients with suppressed immune systems, CMV can produce serious illness. Preterm infants and infants receiving immunosuppressant therapy for transplants are especially at risk. The infection can lead to pneumonia, diarrhea, colitis, liver disease, retinal hemorrhages leading to blindness, and encephalitis. CMV is the leading cause of blindness in HIV-infected patients. Preferred drugs for treating CMV include ganciclovir and foscarnet.

Herpes simplex

Herpes simplex is a chronic infection, which is commonly a reactivation of an earlier herpes infection.

Look for red, blisterlike lesions...

Typical signs include painful red, blister-like lesions occurring in the oral, anal, and genital areas. Vesicles can also be found on the esophageal and tracheo-bronchial mucosa. Other signs and symptoms include pain, bleeding, and discharge.

Treat with acyclovir, famciclovir...

Drugs to treat herpes simplex include acyclovir, famciclovir, and vidarabine.

Herpes zoster

The herpes zoster virus is also known as acute posterior ganglionitis, shingles, zona, and zoster. An acute infection can result from a reactivation of the chickenpox virus.

Look for small, red clusters

Look for small clusters of painful, reddened papules that follow the route of inflamed nerves. The clusters may be disseminated, involving two or more dermatomes, but generally appear on one side of the body.

Treat with acyclovir, famciclovir...

Drugs to treat herpes zoster include acyclovir, famciclovir, valacyclovir, and vidarabine.

Histoplasmosis

Histoplasmosis is a fungal infection that is especially problematic in the southeastern, mid-Atlantic and central United States. It's caused by *Histoplasma capsulatum,* which grows in soil, and it travels by airborne particles to the lungs. It is not transmitted person-to-person.

> Histoplasmosis travels by airborne particles to the lungs. Drat.

Look for fever, weight loss...

Common signs and symptoms of histoplasmosis include fever, weight loss, hepatomegaly, night sweats, productive cough, splenomegaly, and pancytopenia. Less common problems include diarrhea, meningitis, skin lesions, and GI mucosal lesions that result in bleeding.

Treat with amphotericin B

Amphotericin B is the preferred drug to treat histoplasmosis, although fluconazole may be used. After amphotericin B, itraconazole is used as lifelong suppressive therapy.

Mycobacterium avium-intracellulare

Mycobacterium avium-intracellulare (MAI) travels by oral ingestion or inhalation. It can infect the bone marrow, liver, spleen, GI tract, lymph nodes, lungs, skin, brain, adrenal glands, and kidneys. MAI can eventually become chronic. It shows no evidence of person-to-person transmission.

Look for night sweats, abdominal pain...

Signs and symptoms of MAI tend to be multiple and nonspecific. They include fever, night sweats, abdominal pain, chronic diarrhea, lymphadenopathy, hepatomegaly and splenomegaly, anemia, leukopenia, and thrombocytopenia.

Treat with combination therapy

Treat MAI with combination drug therapy: azithromycin or clarithromycin and ethambutol, plus one or more of clofazimine, rifabutin, and rifampin.

Pneumocystis carinii pneumonia

Pneumocystis carinii causes the protozoal infection *Pneumocystis carinii* pneumonia (PCP). PCP is the most common opportunistic infection associated with AIDS. Fortunately, cases are starting to decline with the advent of highly active antiretroviral therapy. The parasite lodges in human lungs and is transmitted by airborne exposure.

> PCP, the most common AIDS-related infection, is caused by a parasite that lodges in yours truly.

Look for mild fever, dyspnea...

Signs and symptoms of PCP include mild fever and dyspnea on exertion that may lead to a nonproductive cough or respiratory failure. PCP may be revealed by a chest X-ray that shows diffuse interstitial infiltrates or a gallium scan that shows diffuse bilateral pulmonary disease, a Pao_2 of 70 mm Hg or less, and no signs of bacterial pneumonia.

Treat with prophylactic therapy

Prophylactic therapy may be prescribed to treat PCP when CD4+ counts decrease to 200 or less. Although commonly responsive to therapy, the infection frequently recurs and requires maintenance treatment. Preferred drugs to treat PCP include atovaquone, dapsone, primaquone, co-trimoxazole, trimetrexate, and pentamidine isethionate. Corticosteroids may be used in the acute stages of lung inflammation. (See *Know your pneumonias.*)

Salmonellosis

A weakened immune response increases the impact of *Salmonella,* food- and water-borne bacteria that cause salmonellosis. The bacteria can spread by ingestion, fecal-oral contact, contact with animal carriers or asymptomatic chronic carriers, and inadequately sterilized endoscopic equipment. The organisms are resilient and persist in the environment despite thorough cleaning. Report outbreaks to local health authorities.

A weakened immune response heightens my effect.

Look for fever, chills...

Signs and symptoms of salmonellosis include fever, chills, weight loss, anorexia, abdominal cramping, and diarrhea.

Know your pneumonias

Along with *Pneumocystis carinii* pneumonia, other pneumonias may appear in HIV-infected patients. Common AIDS-related pneumonias include:

- *Haemophilus*
- *Legionella*
- lobar
- mycoplasmal
- nosocomial.

Haemophilus pneumonia

This type of pneumonia is caused by the *Haemophilus influenzae* virus. Symptoms include fever, sore throat, and respiratory difficulties. Treatment involves ampicillin or third-generation cephalosporins (such as ceftriaxone or cefotaxime). Because *Haemophilus* pneumonia may occur as a secondary infection in patients with HIV, *H. influenzae* type B vaccine is recommended.

Legionella pneumonia

This type of pneumonia is caused by the bacteria *Legionella pneumophila*. Symptoms include low-grade fever, nonproductive cough, GI disturbances, and shortness of breath. Drug therapy may include erythromycin or quinolones. Rifampin or ciprofloxacin may be added to erythromycin.

Lobar pneumonia

This type of pneumonia is caused by the bacteria *Streptococcus pneumoniae*. It commonly occurs in patients with preexisting respiratory illness. Symptoms include fever (temperature above 102° F [39° C]), and rusty sputum production. Treatment may include

(continued)

Know your pneumonias *(continued)*

penicillin G, cefazolin, or erythromycin. This condition commonly occurs in HIV-infected patients with impaired production of specific antibodies.

Mycoplasmal pneumonia

This type of pneumonia is caused by the bacteria *Mycoplasma pneumoniae.* Symptoms include headache, malaise, low-grade fever, sore throat, and dry, paroxysmal cough. Treatment may include erythromycin, tetracycline, or doxycycline.

Nosocomial pneumonias

Pneumonia is one of the most common nosocomial infections. Bacteria that cause nosocomial pneumonia include *Pseudomonas aeruginosa* and *Staphylococcus aureus.* Symptoms include abnormal chest X-ray, change in sputum, and fever. Drug therapy is based on the identified organism from a sputum culture.

Treat with ciprofloxacin, co-trimoxazole...

Treatment for salmonellosis depends on the particular organism but may include ciprofloxacin, cefotaxime, and co-trimoxazole.

Toxoplasmosis

Caused by the parasite *Toxoplasma gondii,* toxoplasmosis may be transmitted by the oral-fecal route or by ingestion of undercooked meats and vegetables. The parasite can also occur in pet feces and become airborne, posing a danger to HIV-positive pet owners. It's rarely acquired from blood products or organ transplantation. The infection may cause brain abscesses, diffuse encephalopathy, and meningoencephalitis.

Look for changes in mental status

Look for changes in the patient's mental and neurologic status, as well as fever.

Treat with sulfadiazine, clindamycin...

Drugs used to treat toxoplasmosis include sulfadiazine, clindamycin, and pyrimethamine with leucovorin.

Tuberculosis

Tuberculosis is a bacterial infection caused by *Mycobacterium tuberculosis*. This organism is spread by inhaling droplet nuclei that are aerosolized by coughing, sneezing, or talking. Report outbreaks to local health authorities.

Droplet nuclei are aerosolized by coughing, sneezing, or talking.

Look for fever, fatigue...

Signs and symptoms of tuberculosis include fever, night sweats, fatigue, dyspnea, chills, hemoptysis, chest pain, and weight loss.

Treat for 6 months or longer

Drug therapy for tuberculosis may include several of the following: isoniazid, rifampin, pyrazinamide, ethambutol, capreomycin, cycloserine, and streptomycin. Drug therapy continues for 6 months or longer until negative sputum cultures occur.

Cancers

The most common cancers associated with HIV are cancer of the cervix, Kaposi's sarcoma, and CNS lymphoma.

Cancer of the cervix

Papanicolaou (Pap) tests may fail to detect cancer of the cervix in an HIV-positive woman. If symptoms suggest cancer of the cervix, the patient should undergo a colposcopy. Most HIV-infected women with cervical cancer die as a result of the cancer, rather than AIDS.

Look for vaginal bleeding, pelvic pain...

Signs and symptoms of cancer of the cervix include:

• in early disease — abnormal vaginal bleeding; dark, foul-smelling vaginal discharge; and postcoital pain and bleeding.

• in advanced stages — pelvic pain, hematuria, anemia, vaginal leakage of urine and feces from a fistula, anorexia, weight loss, and fatigue.

Treat with chemo, radiation...

Treatment for cancer of the cervix includes chemotherapy, radiation, and surgery.

Kaposi's sarcoma

The most common cancer associated with AIDS, Kaposi's sarcoma affects endothelial tissue, which compromises all blood vessels. Classic Kaposi's sarcoma is a rarely fatal disease found predominantly in older men of Mediterranean descent that causes a nonaggressive form of skin cancer. However, AIDS-associated Kaposi's sarcoma is an aggressive form of angiosarcoma (a malignant cancer arising from vascular endothelial cells) that most commonly affects HIV-infected men. Kaposi's sarcoma rarely occurs in women.

Kaposi's sarcoma is the most common AIDS-related cancer.

Look for red-purple lesions

Kaposi's sarcoma can cause external lesions to appear on the face, neck, arms, and legs. It commonly produces red-purple circular lesions that may appear slightly raised. AIDS-associated Kaposi's sarcoma eventually invades the internal organs and tissues, especially those of the GI tract. Kaposi's sarcoma is diagnosed by biopsy.

Treat with chemotherapy...

Chemotherapy is the preferred treatment for deep lesions, although radiation may also be used.

> The risk of malignant lymphoma increases the longer a person survives with AIDS.

Malignant lymphoma

Believed by researchers to stem from a virus, the risk of malignant lymphoma increases the longer a person survives with AIDS. More than 90% of cases are extra-nodal, commonly occurring in the CNS.

Look for a rapidly enlarging mass

A common sign of malignant lymphoma is a rapidly enlarging

mass. Other signs include unexplained
fever, night sweats, or weight loss
greater than 10%. It's diagnosed through
bone marrow biopsy, lumbar puncture,
and mass biopsies.

Treat with chemo, interferon...

Treatment for malignant lymphoma includes chemotherapy, radiation, and the
use of biologic-response modifiers, such
as interferon and colony-stimulating factors.

Primary CNS lymphoma

Primary CNS lymphoma is rare but deadly. People with this cancer have a life expectancy of 4 months.

Look for confusion, lethargy...

Signs and symptoms of primary CNS
lymphoma include confusion, lethargy,
changes in personality or behavior, hemi-
paresis, seizures, headache, and increased intracranial pressure.

Treat with radiation

Surgical treatment for primary CNS
lymphoma remains impractical, and
chemotherapy typically fails to improve

the patient's condition. Radiation provides some relief from symptoms but doesn't improve the patient's overall life expectancy. Patients who haven't had a prior opportunistic infection are more likely to benefit from radiation therapy.

Late complications

When a patient becomes severely immunocompromised, HIV-related complications become more difficult to withstand. AIDS dementia complex and HIV-AIDS wasting syndrome usually occur in end-stage AIDS. Treatment is usually futile.

> AIDS dementia complex occurs in patients with very weak immune systems.

AIDS dementia complex

Also called HIV encephalopathy, AIDS dementia complex occurs in patients with extremely compromised immune systems (CD4+ counts less than 50). The severity of symptoms depends on the extent of CNS destruction. It's the most common neurologic disorder associated with AIDS. This type of dementia differs from dementia caused by oth-

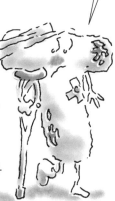

er syndromes in that patients don't have a decreased level of alertness.

The cause of AIDS dementia complex remains unknown. Researchers suspect that HIV-infected macrophages produce neurotoxins that destroy glial cells, the supporting structures of the brain and spinal cord.

Look for confusion, hallucinations, loss of coordination...

Examples of early-stage symptoms of AIDS dementia complex include short-term memory loss, delusions, hallucinations, paranoia, impaired handwriting, leg weakness, and loss of coordination.

Examples of late-stage signs and symptoms include circumlocution, confusion, disinhibition, global dementia, organic psychosis, and coma.

In AIDS dementia complex, the severity of symptoms depends on the extent of CNS destruction.

Treat with psychotropic drugs

Psychotropic drugs can manage behavior, but don't serve as a treatment for AIDS dementia complex. Supportive and symptomatic treatments are the only options.

HIV-AIDS wasting syndrome

The exact cause of HIV-AIDS wasting syndrome is unknown. It may be due to massive, persistent diarrhea. The patient develops severe anorexia and cachexia that prove resistant to weight-gaining efforts.

HIV-AIDS wasting syndrome leads to prolonged hospitalization and a range of complications. It commonly causes malnutrition, functional impairments, and organ dysfunction. It may also compound the adverse effects of drug therapy and cause drug toxicities. Patients who fall below 66% of their ideal body weight face increased risk of death.

Look for weight loss, weakness...

HIV-AIDS wasting syndrome is commonly characterized by:
• involuntary weight loss of 10% or more
• chronic diarrhea for greater than 30 days
• documented fever and weakness of 30 days or greater
• loss of lean body tissue that is disproportional to loss of adipose tissue.

There is no direct test to diagnose HIV-AIDS wasting syndrome. Diagnosis oc-

curs by ruling out other possible causes
of the symptoms.

Treat with appetite enhancers and added nutrition

Treatment for HIV-AIDS wasting syndrome includes appetite-enhancing
drugs and nutritional supplements.

Quick quiz

1. The most common AIDS-related infection is:

    A. herpes zoster.

    B. *Pneumocystis carinii* pneumonia.

    C. salmonellosis.

Answer: B. *Pneumocystis carinii* pneumonia, a protozoan infection, is the most
common AIDS-related opportunistic infection. It's also known as PCP.

2. Kaposi's sarcoma is most likely to occur in:

    A. HIV-positive females.

    B. HIV-positive males.

    C. any HIV-positive patient, regard-
less of sex.

Answer: B. Kaposi's sarcoma is most common in males. It rarely occurs in females.

Scoring

☆☆☆ If you answered both questions correctly, super! Your knowledge is spreading rapidly.

☆☆ If you answered fewer than two questions correctly, it's okay. A review of the chapter usually provides effective treatment.

6

Teaching patients with AIDS

Key facts
- Your teaching should include an explanation of the difference between being HIV-positive and having AIDS.
- Make it clear to the patient that combination antiretroviral therapy has been very successful in minimizing the presence of HIV, but doesn't kill 100% of the virus.
- When discussing safer sex, you'll need to use a nonjudgmental approach and assess the patient's awareness of risks associated with various sexual behaviors.

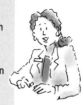

Explaining HIV and AIDS

When teaching patients who've recently been diagnosed HIV-positive, you're likely to hear some common questions

What does being HIV-positive mean?

HIV-positive means that your blood and tissues are infected with the human immunodeficiency virus. HIV is the virus that causes AIDS.

My doctor told me I'm HIV-positive. Does that mean I have AIDS?

Being HIV-positive doesn't necessarily mean you have AIDS. To have acquired immunodeficiency syndrome, or AIDS, you must be infected with HIV, but other criteria must also be met. As HIV infection progresses, the immune system is destroyed. This destruction of the immune system is measured by counting T cells, which help make up the immune system in the body. A T-cell count, also called $CD4^+T$ count, under 200 is one of the criteria for the diagnosis of AIDS.

AIDS isn't one disease. It's a syndrome that can produce more than 26 opportunistic infections or diseases. The presence of one or more of these opportunistic infections or diseases is another criteria for the diagnosis of AIDS.

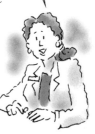

AIDS isn't one disease. It's a syndrome that can produce more than 26 opportunistic infections or diseases.

Can treatment make HIV go away?

At this point, the technology doesn't exist to remove HIV completely from your system. Combination antiretroviral therapy has been very successful in minimizing the presence of HIV in people but doesn't kill 100% of the virus.

Unfortunately, it isn't yet known how long and for whom this combination therapy will work. It's believed that antiretroviral treatment may prevent some patients from getting AIDS or, at least, the treatment can postpone progression to AIDS. Therapies have been available for only a few years, so there are no definite answers. (See *Preventing HIV transmission,* page 118.)

Combination antiretroviral therapy has been successful in minimizing HIV, but doesn't kill 100% of the virus.

Discussing safer sex

When discussing safer sex, use a nonjudgmental approach. Assess the patient's awareness of risks associated with various sexual behaviors. Below are suggested answers to questions patients commonly ask about safer sex.

What is "safer sex"?

Safer sex refers to methods used to reduce the risk of exposure to HIV during sex — for example, placing a condom or other impermeable barrier between the body fluids of one partner and the other. Note the use of the term safer (rather than safe) sex. Nearly all types of sexual behavior carry some risk. (See *Let's talk about sex,* page 120.)

Listen up!

Preventing HIV transmission

To avoid HIV transmission, provide these instructions to your patients:
• If you've been involved in any high-risk sexual activity or have injected I.V. drugs into your body without medical supervision, have a blood test to see if you've been infected with HIV.
• If your blood test is positive or if you take part in high-risk activities and decide not to be tested, inform your sexual partner. If you have vaginal or rectal sex, protect yourself and your partner by wearing a condom correctly from start to finish.
• If your sexual partner has an HIV-positive blood test or if you suspect that your partner has been exposed to HIV, use a condom during sexual intercourse.
• If you or your sexual partner is at high risk, avoid oral contact with the penis, vagina, or rectum.
• Avoid all sexual activities that cause cuts or tears in the lining of the penis, vagina, or rectum.
• Don't have sex with male or female prostitutes. Many prostitutes use I.V. drugs and can infect their clients through sexual intercourse. They can also infect other drug users by sharing I.V. drug equipment. Female prostitutes can also infect their unborn babies.

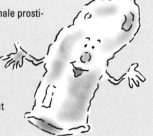

Tell the patient to protect himself and his partner by wearing a condom correctly from start to finish.

What's the best way to avoid HIV infection?

The most effective barrier to HIV and other sexually transmitted diseases is abstinence. If you don't practice abstinence, then maintaining a monogamous relationship with a noninfected partner provides the best protection. Both partners should have two negative HIV tests 3 months apart prior to discussing the possibility of not practicing safer sex.

My partner and I are both HIV-positive. Do we still need to practice safer sex?

When both partners are HIV positive, it remains advisable to practice safer sex. Repeated episodes of unsafe sex can increase the chances of infection with a different strain of HIV, thus attacking the immune system again. (See *Tips for condom use,* page 121.)

Teaching about treatment

Teach the patient that effective self-care for HIV includes managing:
- activity
- diet
- medication.

(Text continues on page 122.)

Listen up!

Let's talk about sex

Describe to your patient the relative risk associated with the following sexual activities.

High-risk practices
• Vaginal or anal intercourse without a condom
• Unprotected oral sex
• Manual anal intercourse
• Oral-anal contact
• Blood contact
• Urine or semen ingestion

Moderate-risk practices
• French kissing
• Anal or vaginal intercourse using nonoxynol-9 and a latex condom
• Fellatio interruptus using nonoxynol-9 and a latex condom
• Cunnilingus using a rubber dam
• Urine contact

Low-risk practices
• Mutual masturbation
• Wearing a latex glove when exploring rectum or vagina
• Closed-mouth kissing
• Massage
• Hugging
• Body-to-body rubbing

Absolutely safe behaviors
• Solitary masturbation
• Fantasy
• Mutually monogamous relationship with a noninfected partner (in which both partners have two negative HIV tests 3 months apart)

Listen up!

Tips for condom use

Provide your patient with these tips for using condoms:

• Use a condom every time you have oral, anal, or vaginal sex.

• Use latex condoms instead of "natural" ones; natural membrane materials, such as lambskin, allow a virus to pass through the pores.

• Open wrappers carefully; a jagged fingernail can tear the condom.

• Lubricate inside the tip of the condom with plain water or a water-based lubricant, such as K-Y jelly, to increase sensation without slippage.

• You can also use spermicidal jelly or foam containing nonoxynol-9, which kills HIV. Don't use oil-based products, such as petroleum jelly, because they can weaken the latex.

• To apply a condom, retract the foreskin, if necessary, and unroll the condom over the entire erect penis. Press out the end of the condom tip to remove air bubbles.

• Add extra water-based lubricant to the outside of the condom before entry. Inadequate lubrication can cause condoms to tear or pull off.

• If the condom begins to slip during intercourse, hold the base with your fingers.

• After ejaculation, hold the condom's base and withdraw before losing the erection.

• Remove the condom with a disposable paper tissue.

• Never reuse a condom.

• Store unused condoms in a cool, dry place because heat can damage the latex.

> Once is enough. Never reuse a condom.

Activity

To reduce the chance of infection, teach the patient to:
• utilize good infection control measures, especially hand washing
• clean up after pets with gloves and a mask
• avoid malls and crowded places during flu and cold seasons
• clean up body secretions using gloves and a bleach and water solution of 1:10
• regularly disinfect the bathroom, telephone, and kitchen counters
• regularly change the kitchen sponge, which is a harbor for infection
• change a toothbrush regularly and after an illness
• avoid sharing personal items such as toothbrushes and razors
• use good-quality filtered water
• get hepatitis A and B vaccinations
• change heating and air conditioning filters regularly.

Diet

Teach the patient the following regarding diet:
• Wash fruits and vegetables thoroughly to avoid infections they may carry.

• Don't eat raw fish, meat, eggs, or shell-fish.
• Follow meat handling precautions placed on the package of raw meat.
• Eat meat that is cooked thoroughly, not rare.
• Follow a bland, low-fiber diet or a diet that doesn't include milk or milk products if GI upset occurs, or if indicated by medication regimen.
• Drink Pedialyte or Gatorade to prevent dehydration from excessive diarrhea.
• Use the food pyramid as a guide to proper nutrition.
• Boost calorie intake with such foods as peanut butter and liquid nutritional supplements.
• Eat six small meals throughout the day to help alleviate nausea.
• Eat dry toast or crackers in the morning to counteract nausea.

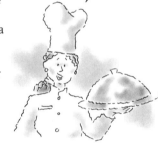

May I recommend some peanut butter and liquid nutritional supplements to boost your calorie intake?

Medication

Teach the patient the following about medication:

- how to properly administer medication, including time, frequency, route, and dosage
- whether medication should be taken with food
- how to recognize signs and symptoms of possible adverse reactions, and the importance of reporting them
- how to take medication consistently to help maintain a prolonged effect
- to wait until after meals, if possible, to take medication that produces nausea
- to prepare a written schedule, listing all drugs and when they should be taken
- to adjust the medication schedule to match his sleeping patterns and his mealtimes.

Long-term concerns

For patients who are HIV-positive, long-term concerns involve such issues as emotional support and life-sustaining treatment.

Support

HIV and AIDS patients and their families need a great deal of support, whether it be emotional, social, or financial. Although every patient's needs differ, most will benefit from the following measures.

Let it out

Encourage your patient to express his feelings and concerns. Help him through the grieving process so he can learn to cope with his losses.

I just stopped by to say hello

Stop to chat with the patient as much as possible. Encourage his family and friends to touch him, hug him, and help with his care. Be tactful and sensitive when gathering personal data.

With a little help from my friends

Encourage the patient to join an HIV support group. Be ready to help him make the initial contact.

Your own two feet

Encourage the patient to be as independent as possible so he can feel he has some control over his condition. Include him in all decision making.

For the down times

If the patient seems severely depressed, discuss antidepressant therapy with the patient, family, and health care provider.

Be flexible

Arrange for flexible visiting hours so family and friends can spend as much time as possible with the patient.

Right on

Advise the patient of his rights. Tell him he has the right to choose what type of treatment he wants, to have procedures explained to him, and to have the privacy and the confidentiality of his medical information maintained.

Lend a hand

If the patient needs financial assistance, refer him to a social worker or a community referral service such as:

• *CDC National AIDS Prevention Information Network.* Go to the Web site (www.cdcnpin.org), then to "databases," then to "resources and services," then search by state or organization; or call (800)458-5231, Monday through Friday, 9 a.m. to 6 p.m. EST.

• *Project inform.* Go to the Web site (www.projinfo.org); or call (800)822-7422, Monday through Friday, noon to 8 p.m.; Saturday, 1 p.m. to 7p.m. EST.

Hop on the hotline

Refer your patient to the National AIDS Hotline, a service of the Centers for Disease Control and Prevention. The National AIDS Hotline is the primary HIV-AIDS information, education, and referral service for the United States. The toll free number is (800)342-AIDS (2437). (For more information on sources of support for AIDS patients, caregivers, and health care providers see *AIDS information online,* pages 128 to 130.)

Life-sustaining treatment

HIV-positive patients may require life-sustaining treatment as they typically suffer a number of medical crises before succumbing to AIDS. For this reason, you'll need to gently discuss the following resuscitation issues with your patient.

Make it clear

Explain the meaning of resuscitation and advanced life support. Tell the patient

(Text continues on page 131.)

AIDS information online

Listed below are several Web sites offering information about AIDS and HIV.

AIDS Clinical Trials Information Service

http://www.actis.org

This site provides easy access to information on federally and privately funded clinical trials. It has links to clinical trial databases, vaccine information, and other resources. You'll find this site helpful if you are looking for general or technical information about the research relating to a specific treatment.

AIDS Treatment News Internet Directory

http://www.aidsnews.org/aidsnews/index.html

Designed for patients and health care professionals, this site is a good starting point for finding credible HIV-AIDS information. The site contains a list of links to other Web sites, organized by topic. The links point to AIDS organizations, calendars of events, reference materials, and other information.

American Foundation for AIDS Research

http://www.amfar.org

The American Foundation for AIDS Research (AmFAR) is a national nonprofit organization created to support AIDS research. This site provides information about AmFAR and the research it funds. You will find this site helpful if you're looking to apply for a grant or participate in one of AmFAR's studies.

American Red Cross

http://www.redcross.org/hss/hivaids

Designed primarily as an educational resource for the general public, this site provides basic information about AIDS. It also includes infor-

AIDS information online *(continued)*

mation on products and services available from the Red Cross, including programs for offices, communities, and schools. You'll find this site helpful if you want to develop an AIDS awareness program.

Association of Nurses in AIDS Care

http://www.anacnet.org/aids

The Association of Nurses in AIDS Care (ANAC) is a national, nonprofit organization for nurses who work with AIDS patients. Along with information about the organization, the Web site provides an online application form. This site is good for nurses who would like additional support from their colleagues.

The Body

http://www.thebody.com

This Web site is an HIV-AIDS information resource containing a 20,000-document library of in-depth information on every stage of diagnosis and treatment. Recommend this site to any patient with HIV or AIDS who wants detailed information about the condition.

Centers For Disease Control and Prevention

http://www.cdc.gov/nchstp/hiv_aids

The Centers for Disease Control and Prevention (CDC) offers general information on a wide variety of diseases, including HIV-AIDS. This Web site is useful if you're looking for HIV-AIDS-related publications, news releases, or referrals.

CDC National Prevention Information Network

http://www.cdcnpin.org

Sponsored by the CDC, this organization was formerly known as the National AIDS Clearinghouse. This site provides thousands of links to HIV-AIDS Web sites, organizations, and publications. Updated daily, this site provides an incredible amount of information.

(continued)

AIDS information online (continued)

Gay Men's Health Crisis
http://www.gmhc.org
Based in New York City, Gay Men's Health Crisis is the oldest and largest nonprofit AIDS organization in the U.S. It supplies aid for local HIV patients and their families while providing education and advocacy worldwide.

HIV/AIDS Treatment Information Service
http://www.hivatis.org
This Web site provides information about federally approved treatment guidelines for HIV and AIDS. The Web site is helpful for people seeking information on the latest clinical trials. Information is available in English and Spanish.

Journal of the American Medical Association
http://www.ama-assn.org/special/hiv
The Journal of the American Medical Association (JAMA) HIV/AIDS Information Center created this Web site as a resource for doctors and other health care professionals. JAMA editors and staff maintain this site with the help of leading HIV-AIDS authorities. Use this site to find the latest clinical information.

National Library of Medicine
http://sis.nlm.nih.gov/hiv.htm
This site provides a massive amount of information, including tutorials on researching HIV-AIDS, information on HIV-AIDS training and outreach programs; and publications, such as fact sheets, manuals, and bibliographies. There are also links to other sites. This is an excellent site for professional research.

that it's his right to decide what life-sustaining measures he wants.

Reassure the patient that being allowed to "die naturally" doesn't mean the end of pain control, comfort measures, or emotional support.

Get it in writing

Emphasize to the patient the importance of documenting his wishes regarding life-sustaining treatment in a living will. A living will is a witnessed document indicating a patient's desire to be allowed to die a natural death rather than be kept alive by heroic life-sustaining measures. The will applies to decisions that will be made after a terminally ill

> If you decide to forgo heroic lifesaving measures, you'll still be provided with pain control, comfort measures, and emotional support.

patient is incompetent and has no reasonable chance of recovery.

In addition, durable power of attorney for health care statutes enable the patient to designate a proxy to make health-related decisions for him if he becomes incompetent.

Considering a companion

If your patient is homosexual, he should be aware that the courts usually don't recognize homosexual relationships. If he wants his companion to act on his behalf, he must have the companion appointed as his legal guardian. Refer the patient to gay and lesbian community services or to a legal agent for legal advice.

Quick quiz

1. Reducing risk in sexual relations involves all of the following except:

A. good communication.
B. latex condoms.
C. natural membrane condoms.

Answer: C. Natural membrane condoms don't protect against viruses or pregnancy.

2. It's unsafe for a patient with AIDS to eat:

    A.   caesar salad with anchovies.
    B.   oysters on the half-shell.
    C.   all of the above.

Answer: C. Both of these foods are capable of spreading food-borne infections.

3. To clean up a blood spill in the home, the patient could use all of the following items except:

    A.   a scrub brush which is then washed in hot, soapy water before reuse.
    B.   1:10 solution of bleach and water, which is then washed down the drain.
    C.   gloves, which are then placed in a disposal container.

Answer: A. A scrub brush would need to be disposed of after this use.

4. A common household item responsible for harboring microorganisms is:

    A.   a toothbrush.

    B.   a kitchen sponge.

    C.   all of the above.

Answer: C. Both of these items can harbor microorganisms.

Scoring

☆☆☆   If you answered all four questions correctly, stupendous! Your skills as a teacher are soaring.

☆☆   If you answered three questions correctly, fabulous! You're ready to communicate with confidence.

☆   If you answered fewer than three questions correctly, don't dodge the classroom. Teachers and students can both benefit from additional review.

Appendix and Index

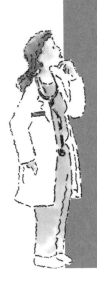

Conditions that define AIDS

The Centers for Disease Control and Prevention (CDC) groups AIDS-related conditions into three categories: A, B, and C. Here's a partial list of AIDS-related conditions classified according to CDC guidelines.

Category A

Persistent, generalized lymph node enlargement or acute (primary) HIV infection with accompanying illness or history of acute HIV infection

Category B

Bacillary angiomatosis, oropharyngeal or persistent vulvovaginal candidiasis, fever or diarrhea lasting more than 1 month, idiopathic thrombocytopenic purpura, pelvic inflammatory disease (especially with a tubo-ovarian abscess), and peripheral neuropathy

Category C

Candidiasis of the bronchi, trachea, lungs, or esophagus; invasive cervical cancer; disseminated or extrapulmonary coccidioidomycosis; extrapulmonary cryptococcosis; chronic intestinal cryptosporidiosis; cytomegalovirus (CMV) disease affecting organs other than the liver, spleen, or lymph nodes; CMV retinitis with vision loss; encephalopathy related to HIV; herpes simplex involving chronic ulcers or herpetic bronchitis, pneumonitis, or esophagitis; disseminated or extrapulmonary histoplasmosis; chronic intestinal isosporiasis; Kaposi's sarcoma; Burkitt's lymphoma or its equivalent; immunoblastic lymphoma or its equivalent; primary brain lymphoma; disseminated or extrapulmonary *Mycobacterium avium* complex or *M. kansasii;* pulmonary or extrapulmonary *M. tuberculosis;* and any other species of *Mycobacterium* (disseminated or extrapulmonary); *Pneumocystis carinii* pneumonia; recurrent pneumonia; progressive multifocal leukoencephalopathy; recurrent *Salmonella* septicemia; toxoplasmosis of the brain; wasting syndrome caused by HIV

Index

i refers to an illustration; t refers to a table.

i refers to an illustration; t refers to a table.

i refers to an illustration; t refers to a table.

i refers to an illustration; t refers to a table.

i refers to an illustration; t refers to a table.

i refers to an illustration; t refers to a table.

i refers to an illustration; t refers to a table.

i refers to an illustration; t refers to a table.